Overcoming M

How changing your lifestyle can change your life

Mark Knoblauch, PhD

Kiremma Press
Houston, TX

ISBN: 978-1-7320674-7-9

Disclaimer: This book is not intended as a substitute for the medical advice of licensed physicians. The reader should regularly consult their physician in matters relating to his/her health and particularly with respect to any symptoms that may require diagnosis or medical attention.

Reviewers:
Ann Svendsen-Sanchez, MS
University of Houston

Jeffrey Vrabec, MD
Otolaryngology-Head & Neck Surgery
Baylor College of Medicine

Penny Wilson, PhD, Registered Dietician Nutritionist
www.eatingforperformance.com

Book Cover and Book Design by AuthorPackages.com

Printed in the United States of America
First Printing March 2018

Publisher: Kiremma Press, Houston TX
Author Website: www.authorMK.com

To my wife, who was there throughout my Ménière's battle, and who has never once doubted the effects nor complained about the required adjustments.

Table of Contents

Foreword

Dr. Mark Knoblauch has prepared a book for Ménière's disease patients by a Ménière's disease patient. The description of the symptoms from the patient perspective and its impact on day to day activities accomplishes his goal of bringing the reader (whether patient, physician, or family member) into the experience of vertigo. While the physical experience of the vertigo may be reproduced by excessive alcohol ingestion, (there are dramatic effects of alcohol on the vestibular organs) Mark correctly explains the two most disturbing factors for the Ménière's patient; he didn't intentionally cause the vertigo and he didn't know when it was going to occur.

The anxiety he experiences at the onset is presented in exquisite detail. With any new diagnosis, there is tremendous uncertainty as to the long-term consequences. The fear is only heightened by misinformation from casual sources. The difficulty in determining where the symptoms are coming from often leads to frustration with the medical community. Numerous physicians may be consulted before ultimately arriving at the ear specialist. The reader senses his exasperation when he feels that no one seems to understand what he is describing.

My job as a Neurotologist is to live the treatment of Ménière's disease. Your primary physician may see this diagnosis a few times per year, in my field I see it daily. I read (and write) the medical literature on Ménière's disease. I attend meetings and discuss this with other Neurotologists nationwide and internationally. We share our experience treating patients and debate the optimal strategy. We collectively share the frustration of not being able to prescribe a medication and watch the patient's symptoms disappear. No, Ménière's disease is far more complex than that. However, rest assured that there are many very bright minds spending their careers attacking the mechanisms of the disease.

Chapter 8 provides an overview of treatments and their effects. Dr. Knoblauch emphasizes the lack of definitive evidence for most treatments and the variability in response. Some treatments work for some patients and not for others. One of the most challenging aspects to the study of various treatments is that the vertigo episodes subside over time. Control groups (untreated subjects) often improve on their own; thus, the effect of any medication is less certain. In contrast, hearing typically declines and no treatment has yet shown the ability to arrest progression of hearing loss.

Ultimately the individual's response to the disease is paramount to treatment success. Dr. Knoblauch refuses to let the disease control his life. He recognizes the impact of lifestyle changes on stress reduction and elimination of anxiety. Reducing stress removes one of the notable triggers for the symptoms. The symptoms will become more predictable and more manageable. I commend his effort to present his experience with Ménière's disease and his ability to overcome the symptoms.

Jeffrey T Vrabec MD
Neurotologist

Introduction

Imagine opening your eyes to see nothing but gray streaks zigzagging back and forth. Imagine trying to stand up after getting out of a chair, only to find that you roll over sharply with no ability to stop yourself from crashing into whatever it is your momentum is carrying you towards. Imagine fearing the day within seconds of waking up, only to beg for nightfall so that you can crawl into bed. Imagine going through each day living in fear of being incapacitated for three or four hours during a violent vertigo attack. And now imagine that this goes on day after day. That is the life for many Ménière's sufferers.

I know all of this because I was one. For over three years my life was dictated by something beyond my control. I would try to ignore it, only to be forcefully reminded of its presence time after time. Cancelations became more frequent. Social events became feared. Physician visits brought no relief, instead only the suggestion that it was all in my head and that I needed to try to relax more. Eventually, a casual conversation led me to a specialist that was able to diagnose me with Ménière's. The diagnosis finally allowed me to target the underlying issue, which in turn led me down the path of a relatively simple low-sodium lifestyle modification that has effectively eliminated my Ménière's symptoms for over six years.

Since you are reading this book I'm guessing that either you have Ménière's disease, you are close to someone who has the disease, or you work with Ménière's patients. If you have Ménière's, you will probably relate well to many aspects in my own journey with Ménière's. For those of you who are close to or work with someone who has Ménière's, this book is designed to help you understand more about this miserable disease.

Back in my symptomatic days, I found several Ménière's-related books but quickly realized that they lacked much of what I wanted to know about the disease. Were my symptoms worse than theirs, the same, or better? What was effective for them? What do we know about the causes of Ménière's? How or why does Ménière's happen? These were questions that I walked away with to some degree for each book I looked through. So, I decided that I would write my own book to put answers to all of my questions into one book.

Therefore, this book is designed to both provide you relevant information about Ménière's disease as well as outline how I was able to effectively eliminate my Ménière's symptoms. The book starts out with a general overview of the anatomy of the ear so as to orient you to the structures that will be discussed in detail in Chapter 2. Next, recent (as of press time) literature is discussed specific to outlining what Ménière's is and how it is thought to be involved with the various parts of the vestibular system. I then introduce you to my own Ménière's story so that you can see the development and struggles I had with Ménière's. Because a relatively simple lifestyle modification has been so successful for me, I then introduce you to sodium to outline what it is, why it is important for the body, and what dietary adjustments were successful for me. We will then conclude with a look at Ménière's treatment options along with other medical conditions of the vestibular system that present similar to Ménière's, followed by a look at how Ménière's can affect an individual's quality of life.

Chapter 1
Anatomy of the Ear

L ET'S FACE IT, MOST of us take our ears for granted. Unless we have some unexpected issue with our hearing we are relatively oblivious to the work that our ears perform. If we cannot hear someone's initial conversation, our first instinct is likely to accuse them of not speaking loudly enough. The problem, however, may lie in the fact that our ears failed to accurately process the incoming sound waves and convert them over to a neurological signal capable of being interpreted by our brain. Accurate processing of sound requires a precise series of events that involves the outer, middle, and inner ear working together as a cohesive unit.

Hearing is essential to our daily activities of living, but our ears do so much more than capture and convert sound waves. Deep within the ear, specialized receptors detect our movement and provide feedback about the position of our body. Our brain's interpretation of these signals allows us to make postural changes necessary to maintain our balance as well as sense our body's position. Complications that affect the inner ear result in a variety of medical conditions including Ménière's disease. Because the structures of the ear are so involved in Ménière's, it is important that in a book about Ménière's we first outline the general anatomy of the ear. We'll take a quick trip through the outer and middle ear before focusing on the inner ear, which houses the vestibular system that is highly involved with Ménière's. Particular focus will be placed on outlining those structures that detect and process balance and motion, along with an overview of the fluid containment system of the ear.

Main sections of the ear

Outer ear

The ear is comprised of three main sections – the outer ear, middle ear, and inner ear (Figure 1.1). The outer ear is effectively that portion of the ear that we can access, consisting of skin and cartilage and continuing down the ear canal to the tympanic membrane, or "eardrum". The outer ear's predominant function is to collect and funnel sound waves to the middle ear. Generally speaking, very little activity transpires along the structures of the outer ear, especially relating to Ménière's or other vestibular disorders.

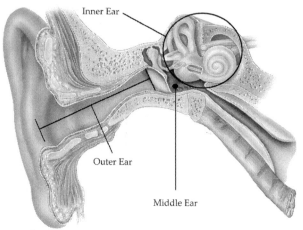

Figure 1.1 The outer, middle, and inner ear compartments each perform highly specialized functions for hearing, balance, and movement detection

Middle ear

The middle ear, along with its inner-ear neighbor, is housed entirely within the temporal bone of the skull. The middle ear comprises the air-filled cavity found internal to the eardrum. Here, the incus, malleus, and stapes bones transfer vibrations from the eardrum to the inner ear where they are then transmitted to the brain.

Inner ear

The inner ear is housed within the temporal bone and includes two main sections – the cochlea and the labyrinth (Figure 1.2).

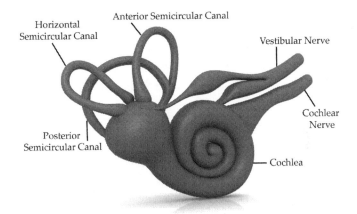

Figure 1.2. The highly sensitive middle ear detects and transmits information to the brain regarding motion and equilibrium as well as head position and movement

Cochlea

The cochlea is a fluid-filled container which holds thousands of hair cells that are connected via nerve cells to the brain. These hair cells are bathed in a potassium-rich fluid called endolymph. Vibrations from the eardrum are transmitted by way of the middle ear bones to the cochlea. There, the vibrations are detected by cochlear hair cells which then convert the vibrations into a neural signal by way of the organ of Corti.

The hair cells of the cochlea are highly sensitive and are therefore subject to damage from a variety of causes such as loud noise, antibiotic medication, or certain diseases such as meningitis. Damage to cochlear hair cells is particularly unfortunate as they are unable to regenerate. Consequently, any cochlear hair cells damaged beyond repair permanently decrease the number of working hair cells.

Vestibular system

The second component of the inner ear is the labyrinth. Here lies the vestibular system which is responsible for detecting body movement and position in addition to aiding in the regulation of balance. The vestibular system consists of three areas – the saccule, utricle, and semicircular canals.

The position of the saccule and utricle allow them to detect linear motion of the head. Forward and backward motion is predominantly detected by the utricle, while vertical motion is detected by the saccule. Within both the saccule and utricle is a structure called the macula that detects and transmits information specific to the head's movement. The interior of each macula is covered by a gelatinous liquid embedded with small calcium-based crystals called *otoliths*. As the head moves, the weight and consequent motion of the otoliths generates inertia. This inertia is detected by hair cells located within the gel, which then send a signal to the brain via an attached nerve specific to the direction of head movement.

While the utricle and saccule detect forward/backward along with vertical movement, the function of the semicircular canals is to detect 'angular' movement. For example, if the head remains stationary while the body is spun around, macula may not detect the motion due to a lack of inertia generated by the otoliths. However, the position of the semicircular canals can detect this motion. The three semicircular canals (termed horizontal, anterior, and posterior) are positioned so that any plane of movement by the head can be detected. The horizontal canal is positioned to best detect side-to-side movement, while the posterior canal detects up-and-down movement such as would occur when nodding. The anterior canal detects side-to-side tilting, such as if the ear is placed on a shoulder.

While the semicircular canals contain hair cells, unlike the utricle and saccule of the cochlea there are no otoliths naturally present. Instead, as the head rotates in a particular direction, fluid within the associated canal lags temporarily behind. As the fluid within the semicircular canal eventually begins to move, the embedded hair cells detect the motion of the fluid and send a signal to the brain allowing for interpretation of the direction of movement.

Fluid of the inner ear

Both the cochlea and vestibular system contain fluids termed endolymph and perilymph. In the healthy ear, these two fluids run close to each other but must be maintained separate from each other as endolymph contains high levels of potassium compared to the low-potassium makeup of the perilymph. Separation of these two fluids occurs through the membranous labyrinth which forms a 'sac' of sorts that houses each fluid separately such that the endolymph is effectively contained within the surrounding perilymph.

An important organ involved in regulation of endolymph fluid is the endolymphatic sac. This organ, though not well understood, is thought to be involved in regulation of both volume and pressure of the endolymph fluid[1] (Figure 1.3). Normally, endolymph flows to the endolymphatic sac through the endolymphatic duct. If the endolymph cannot flow normally through the duct due to an event such as blockage, endoymphatic hydrops form.

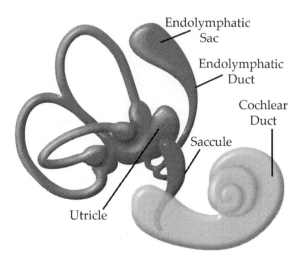

Figure 1.3. The membrane system of the inner ear is responsible for housing and maintaining separation of the fluids found within the intricate labyrinth of the inner ear. Failure of the membrane system to regulate fluid is thought to be a main source of Ménière's disease.

As we will discuss in Chapter 2, endolymphatic hydrops are thought to play a role in Ménière's disease. It is suspected that as hydrops are formed, the resulting increase in endolymphatic pressure causes the membranous labyrinth to break. Upon breakage of the membrane, the separate potassium fluids mix and effectively "confuse" the vestibular nerve receptors that are dependent upon the tight regulation of potassium levels. When the nerve signaling is no longer tightly controlled, the consequent rampant signaling is received by the brain, triggering the symptom of vertigo that is common in Ménière's disease. It is thought that as the membranous labyrinth rupture is repaired, potassium-based fluid levels return to normal and the vertigo symptoms dissipate.

Multiple causes have been proposed as a trigger responsible for the increase in endolymphatic pressure associated with Ménière's. One such theory suggests that there is a defect (i.e. blockage, reduced flow, etc.,) of endolymph into the endolymphatic sac. An alternate theory is that endolymph production is too high, resulting in excess fluid that cannot adequately be removed. Next we will look at these various suspected triggers in more depth in order to better understand the various underlying factors involved in the development of Ménière's. As you will see, much research needs to be conducted in order to conclude or exclude fluid regulation as a contributor to Ménière's.

Summary

The underlying cause of Ménière's disease is not well understood. As such, it remains undetermined as to whether Ménière's results from an alteration or defect of a structure within the ear or if it is due to some other cause such as inflammation or an auto-immune dysfunction. The complexity of the ear lies in part due to the fact that its various organs are involved in both hearing and balance. Given that Ménière's disease can affect the vestibular system along with impacting one's hearing, the possibility exists that the cause of Ménière's lies in a strange combination of factors. At present, the research remains inconsistent in pointing to a likely cause which can make targeted treatment somewhat difficult. Nevertheless, an overwhelming majority of patients respond favorably to Ménière's treatment, indicating that a careful plan should be coordinated between Ménière's patients and their physicians.

Chapter 2
Ménière's Disease

MÉNIÈRE'S DISORDER IS A condition thought to result from problems with the fluid regulation system of the inner ear. Even today, the exact cause of Ménière's is unknown. The symptoms of Ménière's, though, are well documented. Ménière's patients typically experience an ongoing degree of unsteadiness and ear pressure or fullness intermixed with bouts of acute vertigo, nausea, and vomiting that can last several hours.

Most often, Ménière's affects only one ear. However, if Ménière's is discovered at a relatively young age, 50% of those affected in one ear will be affected in the opposite ear within 30 years[2]. In most cases, if the cause of a patient's Ménière's-like symptoms is determined, his or her Ménière's diagnosis is withdrawn and the patient is re-diagnosed under the new condition, as true Ménière's does not have a specific cause. Rather, Ménière's is typically diagnosed after all other possible conditions have been ruled out.

Disease, syndrome, or disorder?

One issue that can invoke confusion is the true classification of

Ménière's. Medical professionals and patients will often describe Ménière's using a variety of terminologies such as Ménière's syndrome, Ménière's disorder, or Ménière's disease. A few decades ago it was proposed that the term *disease* be used for those Ménière's sufferers who have the classic signs and symptoms but an unknown cause. *Disorder* was suggested to be reserved for those patients whose disease cause was known, who had a somewhat incomplete form of the disease, or who are currently under medical evaluation[3]. However, in 2015 a joint commission of several associations released diagnostic criteria for Ménière's *disease*. As such, proper terminology now classifies Ménière's as a disease[4].

The medical origins of Ménière's

Ménière's was first reported in 1861 by Prosper Ménière, a Paris physician. Standard treatment for vertigo and hearing loss at the time was to "bleed" the patient despite little evidence of actual benefit[5]. Ménière himself practiced medicine at Paris' Institute for Deaf-Mutes and had treated numerous patients who developed vertigo after ear trauma. This was significant, as during the time of Prosper Ménière, the understanding of ear function was limited to sound perception; therefore, any abnormalities of balance were attributed to "cerebral congestion". Prosper Ménière was the first to associate balance and dizziness issues with the ear and effectively started the field of vestibular medicine. If you are interested in how Prosper Ménière developed the foundation for our understanding of the inner ear's function, Baloh wrote a detailed academic paper on the subject that makes for an interesting read[5].

Classifying Ménière's

The first official classification of Ménière's disease was presented in 1972 by the American Academy of Otolaryngology-Head and Neck Surgery[6]. At the time, Ménière's was assigned as either "cochlear" or "vestibular", but this separation of Ménière's was eventually abandoned in a later revision released in 1985[7]. Eventually, the AAO-HNS refined the classification of Ménière's disease (MD) into three categories[6]:

* Possible MD: episodic vertigo or fluctuating hearing loss
* Probable MD: one attack of rotatory vertigo lasting at least 20 minutes, together with tinnitus and documented hearing loss
* Definite MD: two or more spontaneous episodes of vertigo 20 minutes or longer with tinnitus and documented hearing loss

The timeline of normal Ménière's can vary from patient to patient, as symptoms can at times be separated by many years and may resemble other conditions of the inner ear. Furthermore, the symptoms associated with Ménière's can fluctuate, disappear, and reappear randomly over time. As such, new criteria were outlined for Ménière's by the Classification Committee of the Barany Society such that two categories were outlined: definite Ménière's disease and probable Ménière's disease[4].

Definite Ménière's disease requires one episodic vertigo syndrome event lasting between 20 minutes and 12 hours, associated with low- to medium-frequency sensorineural hearing loss in the affected ear as well as fluctuating aural symptoms (ear fullness, tinnitus, or hearing issues). Probable Ménière's disease includes episodic vestibular symptoms (e.g. dizziness or vertigo) associated with fluctuating aural symptoms lasting from 20 minutes to 24 hours.

Despite the evolving definitions of Ménière's, the symptoms associated with Ménière's are relatively consistent and include fluctuating hearing loss and tinnitus, episodic vertigo, ear 'fullness' or pressure, instability, nausea, and in some cases "drop attacks". These drop attacks, or "Tumarkin falls", occur in just a small portion of Ménière's patients but are described as the patient being pushed to the ground, often with perceived "tilting" of the surrounding environment[8].

Who is affected?

The prevalence of Ménière's has been reported to range from 190 to 513 cases per 100,000 people[9, 10], though this wide prevalence range has been reported to be due to methodological differences, changing diagnostic criteria of Ménière's, and the similarity between Ménière's and other vestibular conditions, as well as issues with the patients surveyed[11]. Furthermore, prevalence appears to increase with age. Children and adolescents show a prevalence of just 8 in 100,000 while the rate in adults is 440 per 100,000[11] with the onset of Ménière's typically occurring between the patient's fourth and seventh decade. By gender, Ménière's disease shows a higher prevalence in females than males.

Suspected causes

Several underlying causes of Ménière's have been proposed, including water regulation, endolymph reabsorption anomalies, vascular abnormalities, and autoimmune factors[5, 12]. Though none of these potential abnormalities have been universally accepted, one condition known as endolymphatic hydrops (EH) is consistently associated with Ménière's disease.

As detailed in Chapter 1 of this book, endolymphatic hydrops form due to a distention of the endolymphatic space which then enters into the perilymphatic space. Formation of hydrops within the utricle, saccule, and cochlear duct of the inner ear have been shown to nearly triple the volume of the endolymph[13]. Early research with samples of temporal bones – in which the inner ear is located – indicate that nearly all cases of Ménière's were associated with endolymphatic hydrops[14], and this was confirmed more recently in living patients imaged via magnetic resonance imaging

(MRI) as well[15]. However, not all patients found to have EH report symptoms of Ménière's[16]. Furthermore, EH produces relatively inconsistent clinical symptoms.

Interestingly, conflicting reports indicate that in the presence of endolymphatic hydrops, hearing can either remain strong[17] or be diminished[18]. This inconsistent evidence confounds the likelihood of endolymphatic hydrops being the sole cause of Ménière's. Whereas effectively all Ménière's patients have hydrops, coupled with the fact that Ménière's patients lose hearing in the affected ear over time, it would seem logical that patients with hydrops would also lose hearing. However, the fact that this is not the case is evidence that multiple underlying causes contribute to the effects of Ménière's.

Despite an association between endolymphatic hydrops and Ménière's, other findings suggest that additional structures of the ear may play a role. For example, it has been shown that Ménière's patients suffering from drop attacks exhibit significant degeneration of their otolithic membrane[19]. This lends evidence to the fact that some Ménière's patients (i.e. drop attack sufferers) may have an underlying influence from otolith-based organs rather than endolymphatic hydrops. This is not to say that degeneration of the otolithic membrane is the sole cause, as perhaps a link exists between endolymphatic hydrops and otolithic membrane deterioration. Accordingly, deterioration of an organ that plays an important role in balance certainly suggests an involvement.

Fluid regulation in the middle ear is also thought to be involved in Ménière's. Water channels, which regulate transport of water across cell membranes, have been implicated as possible causes of Ménière's[8, 20]. Unexpected reductions or increases in the number of water channels can influence the balance of fluid on each side of a membrane. Similarly, some researchers suggest that Ménière's patients have a diminished capacity to regulate fluid within their inner ear[21]. Consequently, fluctuations in the inner ear fluid are not well tolerated in

Ménière's patients. This is thought to lead to fluid imbalances that contribute to many of the symptoms encountered by Ménière's patients. Electrolytes such as sodium that are known to play a role in the body's fluid regulation are commonly restricted in Ménière's patients in order to reduce potential fluctuations within the middle ear.

There are a wealth of other potential underlying causes associated with Ménière's disease, including autoimmune disorders[22], the herpes virus[23], cervical disorders[24], and stress[25], among others. Whereas no definitive underlying source of Ménière's has been discovered, it is vital that research continues to investigate these and all logical possibilities.

Due in large part to the complexity and sensitivity of the vestibular system, Ménière's remains a complicated disease. During acute attacks Ménière's can be extremely debilitating, followed by months or years of the same individual reporting almost no symptoms. As we will discuss in later chapters, Ménière's treatments that are successful for one individual will often have no effect on many other patients. Or, symptoms exhibited by one Ménière's patient may be relatively absent in another with a more severe form of the disease. These issues have been confounding medical professionals for decades, and while at present there remains no cure for Ménière's, advancements in the field of vestibular medicine lend evidence toward isolating a primary source of Ménière's. When that happens, target treatments will likely follow, thereby improving the opportunity to end the misery for thousands of patients affected by Ménière's.

Chapter 3
My Ménière's Story

The Initial Attack

TO SAY WHEN MY Ménière's symptoms started isn't easy to answer, given the wide variety of symptoms associated with the condition. What I can say with certainty, however, is when I had my first Ménière's attack. It was on a Monday in November of 2008 at 3:30 in the morning. I was literally as inactive as I could possibly be, which is to say that I was asleep. I woke up, confused, feeling miserable and covered in sweat. My plan was to wait it out and deal with it in the morning – but for now I would sleep. It was at that point that I distinctly remember rolling over and having the strangest sensation.

One thing about Ménière's is that many of the symptoms can be extremely difficult to explain. That night, rolling over in bed as I had done thousands of times before, what I first felt was a sort of 'whooshing' sensation similar to if you were in a car turning sharply to one side. I opened my eyes only to find that they weren't working. Well, not working correctly anyway. My vision was beyond blurry, to the point it was more of a bunch of gray streaks resulting from my eyes rapidly moving side to side. When I grabbed my cell phone to check the time I could not read the screen, even while holding it six inches from my face. I'd had mild vertigo before due to congestion, so I decided to wait this one out. Accepting of my fate for the night, I closed my eyes and laid back down to let it pass.

About ten agonizing minutes later I realized I would not be able to remain in bed. A rapidly approaching onset of nausea was arriving and I knew that I had to get to the bathroom located less than ten feet away. I swung the lower half of my body out of bed, stood up, and . . . was quickly slammed sideways against the wall. The vertigo that was evident in bed was now raging, as though standing up had activated a different level. The sweating that had been heavy now grew more profuse.

Even though it was dark, and my eyes weren't working, I tried my best to start towards the bathroom but my legs weren't having it. My vision had now changed such that the room was spinning as if I were stuck on an unfortunate ride. The nausea increased, and I had no choice but to get to the toilet or have a mighty mess on my hands. I moved to my hands and knees, yet the imbalance was prevalent. I had to 'feel' for the floor even while crawling because my brain wasn't processing my movements, forcing me to make wide sweeping motions with my hands and my knees to ensure I was still positioned correctly on the floor. A minute later, just prior to the end result of the nausea arriving, I made it safely into the bathroom.

What happened next was the most incredibly forceful vomiting I had ever experienced. Every successive Ménière's event led to the same thing as that first night - vomiting so vigorous that the next day my upper traps (i.e. shoulder muscles) were sore. I cannot remember this ever happening when I vomited due to normal causes like food poisoning. Even though nothing was coming out, it was as if my body was going to force *something* out, even if that something was my stomach itself. Finally, after a few rounds of retching, my body gave the signal that it was ready to move on.

Throughout the vomiting, I remained covered in sweat. I remember wiping my face off at the toilet and feeling my hair soaked through with sweat. As I looked up from the toilet, the motion of my head brought back the return of that 'whooshing' feeling again. I figured that this had to just be a bad case of food poisoning, so my goal was to get back to bed and let it run its course. I tried to stand up, realized halfway through the process that standing wasn't going to happen, and slowly crawled awkwardly back to bed. Lying down still provided my best recourse, so that's what I did. Although the sweating continued, the sensations of vertigo and the rotary vision seemed less pronounced when I laid still. Finally, after lying through a few more minutes of agony, I fell back asleep.

I've learned that when you have an attack at night, waking up the following morning makes you wonder if it ever happened at all as the symptoms have relatively disappeared. That Monday morning following the first attack I woke up relatively normal. I sat up without a problem, was able to read the clock, and could even stand and walk. My thoughts naturally turned towards whether I had dreamed the incident or if perhaps I was fabricating the events of the night before. Regardless, I showered, got dressed, and headed out the door for an appointment.

By 8:30 in the morning the sun is well on its way across the sky. That morning when stepping out of my relatively dark apartment I was quickly introduced to my newest Ménière's symptom – a vision-related 'haziness' that would follow me for a day or two after an attack. Walking to my car, the air around me seemed to have a sort of haze even though I knew it wasn't truly foggy. The brightness was amplified somewhat; the whites were brighter and bright light was now blinding. I hadn't remembered any of this occurring after my previous congestion-related vertigo episode years before, but I figured it would pass eventually. Until then, I found solace behind a cheap pair of sunglasses.

As I started to drive, I felt an uneasiness. It was as if I wasn't connected firmly to my seat. If I turned the car, my body felt as if it were being pushed excessively farther than the turn warranted. If I stopped, I felt as though I was going to fall forward into the windshield. Somehow my balance wasn't registering correctly with how my body was actually moving. The sensations were tolerable but extremely awkward, and a bit strange to someone who has never experienced them before.

As I arrived at my appointment where I was to inventory a sales representative's supply, I soon realized that thinking – or perhaps calculating – was an extremely taxing process. I learned later that I was experiencing the 'brain fog' effect that follows a Ménière's attack. As I tried to sum up the contents of rows and rows of cases, any variance in the numbers seemed like an unusually difficult challenge. I tried to keep the effects of the brain fog to myself, and I evidently did a good job of covering my struggles up, as I was never asked if I was "ok". As the appointment finished, I headed to my normal duties as a graduate student, and throughout the day noticed that the vision issues as well as the brain fog gradually subsided. The food poisoning event, as I had associated it at the time, was officially gone.

Follow-up attacks

As I mentioned, this first attack happened on an early Monday morning. The preceding Sunday had been rather uneventful as most are for graduate students, but I do know that I had partaken in my weekly Sunday dinner splurge. During my student days I would eat healthy yet cheap during the week – surviving on pasta and rice dishes – then allow myself to splurge a bit on Sundays. The Sunday evening before my attack I had consumed a pack of bratwursts on hoagie buns, topped with barbecue sauce and onions. I had been craving them for a few days but had saved enjoying them until my Sunday feast. At the time, I had little suspicion that my attack had been due to the food, as I had eaten the same meal several times previously.

The rest of the week had gone off without a hitch. Then, the next Sunday night I again had an attack. Not as severe as the first, but severe enough that I was certain that it was another food poisoning issue. I had eaten my 'BBQ sampler', which consisted of chicken legs and summer sausage cooked on the patio grill. Hating my bad luck at having 'food poisoning' two weeks in a row, I started to think that I would need to give up my Sunday treat if it was indeed going to incapacitate me.

Once again, the next day brought a few lingering effects but the vertigo, sweating, and nausea event was gone by the time I woke up Monday morning. The rest of the week went by without incident, until this time I had an attack on the next Monday. It could not be coincidental. I knew that something was up, but diet was the last consideration on my mind. I began thinking more along the lines of severe events such as stroke, seizure, or epilepsy. I scanned the internet for information, but the deeper I got into each condition the more I was convinced that I didn't have that particular condition. This can be somewhat of a relief and yet somewhat frustrating, as eliminating a particular medical condition does not necessarily bring you closer to any kind of answer. Still, I could not find anything that in my mind produced symptoms similar to what I was experiencing.

The next Sunday night brought another attack. My mind was racing as I laid in bed, sweating out what seemed to be half of my body weight. Four attacks on four straight weekends. I specifically excluded food as a trigger, as my whole life I had been eating without incident the same type of foods I was eating now. And, I had eaten different foods prior to each attack. What I didn't know at the time is that while the foods were different, certain characteristics of those foods were the same.

I started to fear the weekend, dreading the next attack. At the same time I began to think about what would happen if these attacks came during work, or while driving. I had tried several times to 'push through' the vertigo and carry on as if nothing was happening, but each time I was either knocked to the ground or found myself quickly seeking out a place to lay down. I wasn't going to win that battle. I had to accept that whenever these strange events hit, I would need to simply wait them out – all three to four hours' worth.

The next thing I knew, I made it through a weekend with no attack. I thought perhaps that 'bug' had passed. And then the next weekend passed. OK, it was gone and I was back to my old self. Unfortunately, this bit of complacency was interrupted two weeks later when the inevitable happened – an attack struck at work. Luckily as a graduate student my schedule was a bit flexible compared to that of corporate life. I didn't *have* to be in a particular place very often. Rather, my life at the time was "get these things done", with the time course of getting things done being somewhat left up to me. So even though the attack happened at work, I was able to find a secluded area with a reclining chair and let the attack have its way with me. It wasn't my worst attack, but the fact that it occurred at my work was somewhat troubling. And the fact that the attacks were starting again was particularly disheartening.

And so it continued. Over the next few months the attacks slowly grew more spread out, but they continued to come at random times. One occurred while playing a game on my phone in bed. One when I leaned forward to focus on something on my computer screen. One while sitting back motionless against the couch watching television. Despite no similarities in my activity at the time of the attack, it was the same sequence of events every time – a sudden shaking sensation in my head, a dropping sensation in my chest, tunnel vision, and a rapid and pounding heart rate. Soon after, the vertigo and profuse sweating would kick in. Ten to 30 minutes after those events started, the nausea would occur before culminating with a round of vomiting.

In between the attacks I noticed that other issues were starting to arise. I felt minor 'whooshing' sensations more often. Turning my head too fast or walking around a corner brought on a brief burst of unsteadiness. Walking down a long straight hallway became physically challenging, at times requiring me to touch a wall. Going down a circular stairwell induced dizziness. I noticed that my vision became shaky, such that if I tried to focus on a tiny object it would seem to be vibrating around. And my right ear fluctuated between producing a low hum and a 'howling' sound, similar to the wind through a tree.

I had noticed for a while that my right ear always felt like it was full, almost as if I were congested just in that ear. My thoughts focused on perhaps an inner ear infection, or maybe a prolonged bout of swimmer's ear, or a ruptured eardrum. My medical training had taught me that balance was largely the responsibility of the ear, so it made perfect sense that my ear would be causing my problems. Eventually, I saw my physician. He looked in my ears and performed a thorough evaluation but found nothing wrong. Dejected, my hopes for an easy explanation were again dashed.

Over the next few months, the symptoms continued along with the attacks. Anticipating the next sudden and severe onset of an attack began to overpower my day, as I had to plan out my schedule 'just in case' an attack hit. I often stayed at home or did things by myself as much as I could. I traveled on city roads rather than freeways so that I could pull off into a parking lot if needed. I drove myself places rather than accepting a ride, in the event that I would have to leave quickly due to an attack. I eventually found myself working diligently to come up with reasons to avoid going with others to public places. If I did ultimately go, I spent my first few minutes analyzing the layout in the event I needed to find a quiet, secluded area to let an attack play out. At minimal, I could not relax until I located the men's bathroom.

They say that men think about sex every 20 seconds. Whether that's true or not is up for debate but I can tell you that it pales in how often I was thinking about my Ménière's. Why? Because at least in my case the reminders – known more commonly as symptoms – were always there. And when you think about the symptoms you start analyzing every one of them, wondering if they are getting worse or better, and if they are getting worse does it mean an attack is imminent. If I stood, I would get dizzy. If I walked, I would become unsteady. I noticed a constant sort of buzzing inside of my head, almost as if there was some kind of low-grade electrical current passing around my brain. Staring at an object cause it to shake back and forth in my vision. Driving induced unsteadiness. It was constant. Ménière's was constant, all day.

I remember that the most relaxed I would feel was crawling into bed at night. There existed my comfort zone. If an attack happened in bed, I was in a safe space and could ride it out. But you can't lay in bed forever. If nighttime brought relaxation, mornings induced stress. Waking up brought three or four seconds of blissful ignorance before my brain woke up and reminded me that not only will I be dizzy all day, but I may or may not have a debilitating three hour vertigo attack. And if an attack doesn't come today, eh, oh well, we'll try again tomorrow. My life was literally being held hostage by my own body.

By the summer of 2010 my frustration seemed to reach an all-time high yet at the same time I had resigned myself to living with this issue the rest of my life. There wasn't much improvement, and the general symptoms were still present all day, every day. Believe me, there's little encouragement in realizing that you are not even statistically halfway through your life yet the remainder of it will be filled with some mysterious condition that brings misery and constant anxiety. I had begun to notice that the frequency of the attacks became more spread out, occurring every month or two. While this was a positive in that they became less frequent, it also induced quite a bit of anxiety as that second month would approach.

The final straw

One early morning in August of 2010 I was sitting at a stop light, waiting for the red left-turn arrow to change to green. I pulled out my phone, flipped it open, and looked down at it. Instantly, a dropping sensation occurred in my chest right as my vision faded, my hearing closed off, and a rapid fit of tunnel vision set in. I immediately shot back in my seat, temporarily paralyzed with fear. A few seconds later, the symptoms began diminishing. The light turned green, and I carefully made my left turn. I immediately turned into a retail pharmacy parking lot. I sat there for a few minutes, leaning into the air conditioner vent to try and derail the oncoming perspiration bout. As I waited, I began to feel as if the event was fading. I rationalized that sitting in the parking lot was doing me no good so I figured I would get back on the road. If my symptoms kept improving I would head to work; if not, I could head back to my apartment since it was on the way.

As I drove, I realized I kept leaning to the right in my car. Then, the 'whooshing' reappeared if I made any head movements, making it difficult to turn my head to look over at my right mirror prior to making a lane change. I decided to head home, where approximately one mile prior to my destination I vomited forcefully. Finally reaching my apartment, I got out of my car and noticed that I was severely listing to my right, causing quite a bit of difficulty in trying to make it up the stairs. Realizing that this was slowly turning into a full-on attack, my mind began reorganizing my daily schedule to account for the three to four hours I was about to miss. As I laid in bed, sweating, begging for the oncoming vertigo to end, a part of me looked forward to the intensely deep sleep that always followed a severe attack. At best, I could now expect to accomplish a couple hours of work that day – if the eventual brain fog would allow it.

About four hours later I woke up and headed in to get some work done in preparation for an experiment I was planning. But something else was on my mind. I was fed up. I sat myself down at my computer and searched for medical forums. If I couldn't figure out the source of my problem, I'd let someone else figure it out for me. Desperate and defeated, I went to a popular website and typed out the events of that morning as well as the general symptoms I had been experiencing. The first responses that came back over the following minutes were quite simply annoying. "That sounds terrible", one stated. Another rambled before finishing with "I will pray for you". At that time, I didn't want prayers, I wanted answers.

The sixth response was longer so I was expecting at least some kind of a legitimate reply. By the second sentence, I had a chill go down my spine. "What you are describing sounds a lot like Ménière's disease". That sentence hit me, because in my trying to find an answer for what was going on I had read about Ménière's but didn't think that I was old enough in my mid-thirties for it to be a likely possibility. In hindsight, I may have been in a fit of denial after having read about the symptoms and its effect on one's life. Still, I didn't want to believe that I had Ménière's, rather hoping that mine was along the lines of labyrinthitis or something whose effects sounded less devastating.

I made another appointment with my physician. I mentioned Ménière's but it didn't register with him as a likely possibility, pointing out that I was statistically too young to have Ménière's. Because the collection of symptoms were becoming almost incapacitating at times – often trapping me at work or home – we began to find a source for my condition. This sent me from a neurologist to a cardiologist, each of which performed several tests over many days, only to find nothing wrong. To this day I cannot decide if being told that they can find nothing wrong is a blessing or a curse, knowing that I am not fine. Every visit I made resulted in yet another doctor unable to help me solve or fix my medical problem. Rather, I was told on more than one occasion to just try and "relax".

As the months drug on, so too did the issues I was having. I began to track patterns in my symptoms, but had very little luck. What I did notice was that my hearing was diminishing in my right ear. Being in an area with a lot of background noise made me effectively deaf as I could no longer isolate one conversation in an area full of sound or other conversations. Yet, on rare occasions, the pressure and loud, low humming sound in my right ear would be almost gone. Any excitement I felt from thinking that my condition was improving would be gone a day or two later upon waking up to again feel the pressure and hear the loud hum. Every morning when I opened my eyes I would stare momentarily at the wall, checking my vision. And every morning I would find that my vision maintained its small, jerky movements. It was a vicious cycle of minor feelings of improvement followed by massive disappointments.

While all of this was going on, life still had to happen. The ongoing symptoms were tolerable, annoying as though they were. The attacks, however, were unbearable and the constant thought of an impending attack nearly drove me insane. My doctor prescribed alprazolam to help, but it was useless and I rarely took a pill. Still, I had my dissertation research to conduct, income to earn (through the inventory appointments), and somehow spend time with my then-fiancé. Unfortunately for each of them, they were always second on my mind. The constant array of symptoms along with the constant fear of an attack is always at the forefront of your thought process. The symptoms literally dictate what you do and when you do it. I couldn't 'push through' an attack, so I had to ensure that I always had a three-hour block of time available in the event an attack hit. And those around me ended up suffering the consequences of that, through missed appointments, canceled dates, and ever-present bouts of agitation.

Other than my ongoing – and as of yet undiagnosed – Ménière's, 2011 was a pretty good year for me. My fiancé and I got married in Florida, I defended my dissertation in which I looked at how cholesterol influences skeletal muscle damage, and I accepted the offer of a post-doctoral fellowship at a major medical college in Houston. Things were going well, except for that constant reminder that I would feel miserable for the rest of my life. In September of 2011 my wife found out she was pregnant, so despite immense joy and excitement, like all joy I felt at the time it was immediately tempered by the depressing reminder of this strange condition I had. But things were about to look up.

Finally, a diagnosis

In the fall of 2011 I was invited to a social gathering with some faculty from my previous institution. Feeling like one of them now, I couldn't pass up the opportunity to socialize with them rather than feel somewhat subservient as I had during my previous years as a mere graduate student. While there, I sat next to one faculty member who had performed balance testing on astronauts and who I had previously talked to about my ongoing issues. I had originally thrown out the word Ménière's to him, but he dismissed it with the rationale that I was too young. That night though, approximately six months after our earlier conversation, he raised the question of how I was feeling. I replied that nothing had changed, and started to tell him again of the recurring symptoms I'd been having. "It was suggested that I have Ménière's", I said, "and I've pretty much resigned myself to that fact". He listened and asked if I had seen an ear specialist. Telling him that I had not yet seen one, he gave me the name of a colleague of his who worked with an ear doctor and told me to send her a quick email.

In my state of despair, I expected yet another fruitless evaluation, but at the same time I was excited at yet another opportunity to figure out what is going on in my head.

The next morning I typed a long email explaining the various issues I'd been having along with all of the unremarkable information I had heard from previous physician evaluations. I outlined the symptoms, the balance issues, and the medications I had tried. About an hour later I received a phone call from her. She described how she worked with a neurotologist, a medical specialty that I had little familiarity with. By the end of that phone call I was more encouraged about getting an answer than at any time previously, yet my enthusiasm was subdued as she told me that it sounds like I may have an inner-ear issue. I knew that Ménière's was an inner-ear problem, and I was dreading that diagnosis after having read about how Ménière's patients have trouble walking in later life, gradually lose their hearing, and can be suicidal – something that I had grown particularly aware of in my own life. Only later would I find out that I was focusing in on the worst of Ménière's, not the most common aspects.

After a quick consult with the physician I was referred to a therapy area where a technician put me through a battery of tests. My thoughts were similar to my expected outcome after all of the testing at both the neurologist and cardiologist – that nothing would be found and I would just be told to 'relax' more. And actually, I was somewhat correct. From some strange clicking device pushed against my ear to cold and hot water swirling in my ear canal to the giant big-top-circus-resembling curtain that was dropped around me, I passed all of the tests. This time, though, it wasn't necessarily unexpected news as those tests check for multiple inner ear, balance, and coordination conditions. Ménière's disease is considered by many to be a condition of exclusion, meaning that when symptoms are combined with certain negative test outcomes, Ménière's is often the diagnosis.

After the testing, I was sent for a hearing check. By the conclusion of the test I knew myself that the results would show a deficiency in my right ear, which the printout clearly showed. In returning for a meeting with the physician, I was slightly enthused that I had passed all of my tests, but still did not have an answer. After a lengthy discussion, the conversation turned to Ménière's. Looking over my results again, he responded with a couple of nods that he feels that I am showing the classic symptoms of Ménière's disease in my right ear. Again feeling a mix of relief and depression, I asked about treatments, triggers, and cures. He outlined everything for me – it was not curable but it is treatable, which in turn led to a discussion of the triggers. I was directed to reduce my sodium intake and limit any potential areas of stress, to which I remember laughing. I am a pretty stress-free individual compared to most. The only stress I had was induced by the Ménière's symptoms. To reduce stress I had to fix Ménière's. Ironically, to fix Ménière's I was instructed to reduce stress. A vicious cycle indeed.

The initial plan was for me to reduce my sodium intake and begin a regimen of two medications – a diuretic along with betahistine. I left the physician's office under mixed feelings. I didn't feel that I consumed a lot of sodium, so I didn't foresee much benefit from that. And, the diuretic wasn't designed to directly affect my ear but rather work to eliminate sodium from my body, so I felt somewhat dejected that I was taking something that wouldn't directly attack the problem in my ear. In hindsight, I realize now how naïve I was regarding my sodium intake specific to my expectations for a cure; however, I also accepted that my ongoing frustrations with my condition were driving my mind to become irrational.

The next few weeks were encouraging. I set out to avoid adding salt to my food, and I passed on any high-sodium food such as sausage, fast food, or soups. I thought back to my very first attack the night after I had eaten the bratwurst and started to think that maybe it was simply a sodium issue. Within a week I noticed that the sometimes humming, sometimes howling sound in my ear was effectively gone, as was the fullness or pressure that had been almost constant. As a result of my ear's improvement, I could suddenly hear better in my right ear as well – almost normal, I asserted. Two weeks later, the jumpiness in my vision disappeared. I noticed that I could walk down a long, straight hallway or around a corner without issue. The unsteadiness I felt on sloped or uneven sidewalks dissipated. And my head just felt 'clearer'.

My enthusiasm for a return to normalcy kept growing. I began to eat more salads, less fried foods, and avoided fast food altogether. My symptoms kept improving. Not fully gone, but improving. The birth of my daughter kept approaching as well, from five, to four, to two months. I began to grow more excited about the prospect of being a dad, and worried less about living with dizziness the rest of my life. Life was improving, and in my mind it was about to become outstanding.

Tick . . . Tick . . . Tick

In mid-May, two weeks before my daughter's due date, I made a pot roast in the slow cooker one Sunday. I hadn't been as diligent about monitoring my sodium simply because as the past few months progressed, I hadn't had the constant reminders of a howling ear, or unsteadiness, or shaky vision. In fact, I had become complacent enough to add a packet of onion soup mix to the pot roast.

The next day, driving home from work I approached a stop light. As I started to slow down, I felt a tremendous "whoosh" that slung my upper body forward. I knew the feeling immediately, which in part led to the rapid increase in heart rate that followed. I turned the corner and made it home, with only some light dizziness due in part to the poor condition of the road that caused my vehicle to bounce around tremendously.

Despite having my guard up, the rest of the evening went without incident. I woke up the next morning and went to work, convinced that the previous day's events were simply a fluke. All was fine through the first half of the day. As I had a one-hour break during an experiment, I decided to walk across the street for lunch as I had done many times previously.

Stepping off a curb and into a main intersection, my sense of normalcy was stolen by the time my foot hit the concrete. I clearly remember my vision becoming a gray blur as my eyes zoomed back and forth rapidly. I immediately fell to the ground in the middle of one of the busiest intersections in the area. A swarm of people came around me as two cars were pulling up to the stop sign that towered over me. "Are you OK?" I was asked at least fifty times. Slowly my vision returned as my eyes slowed, but I could feel the perspiration and vertigo approaching quickly. "I'm fine", I replied. "I just have a little dizzy spell every now and then, and just need to get back to my office. I'll be fine". I had just told multiple lies, but since I already felt like I was in hell, what difference would it make?

I knew I was against the clock. The attack was going to get worse over the next five minutes to the point that the attack would render me unable to walk. And causing one scene in the intersection was bad enough – I didn't want a whole medical college calling a 'code blue' about some crazy guy laying in a hallway. As the perspiration increased, the rotational vertigo started to kick in. It was getting worse. Luckily, my experiment was being conducted in a small room in the basement of the building where I would likely not be disturbed. I had to get to that room. My biggest obstacle was approaching – the damn elevators that either arrive instantly or take five or more minutes. Prayer was not involved much in my Ménière's, but that day one was sent off, asking selfishly for a quick elevator.

As I reached the room, I immediately shut the light off and rolled my chair over to the countertop. I rested my head and elbows on the counter and pulled the trash can underneath me, waiting for the muscle-straining vomiting session. A million things were going through my head, predominantly the anguish of thinking that the attacks were starting up again. As I began to play out what happened, a sort of metronome sound came from below me. Tick – tick – tick. The sound of sweat dripping off of my chin and onto a crumpled up paper bag provided the only sound in the room. Until, that is, ten minutes later when the agonizing vomiting session started.

The events of that afternoon went down as my worst, most violent Ménière's attack to date. And my incident in the street provided me my first experience with the 'drop attacks' inherent to severely affected Ménière's patients. Luckily, I was able to finish my experiment hours later, but my mind was not on science but rather on how I am going to deal with the return of the attacks. I made a quick call to my neurotologist, whose office happened to be just a quarter mile away. My hope was that he could see me immediately and evaluate the after-effects of brain fog and the sensitivity to bright light. Unfortunately for me, he had left for the day. But, I was able to schedule an appointment for the next day.

At 10am the following morning, I cried like a baby. Sitting in the doctor's office, the anguish from the recent attack was still with me. For the first time since I had Ménière's, I cried my heart out. A sobbing, weeping, can't-interpret kind of cry. And I didn't care who witnessed it. I didn't care about anything, quite frankly, including any proposed reason not to put a bullet in my brain. The thoughts in my head had gotten that bad. My first child was going to be born in two weeks and I didn't even care. Over the past few months I thought I had beaten Ménière's, only to have it now return with a vengeance. And I didn't have the mental strength to fight it for the next 40 years. I thought repeatedly about how when someone dies, those around him or her say "finally, they are at peace". I only hoped that my wife would realize that if I were dead, she could somehow accept that I too was at peace. Even though it was a single attack that previous afternoon, the prospect of falling back into the grasp of Ménière's was overwhelming.

When the sobbing stopped I was finally able to explain what happened. The doctor asked a few questions, to which I revealed that I had eaten the roast containing the soup mix. That spurred a discussion about hidden sources of sodium, of which I had not thoroughly been checking. He reiterated the need to take the diuretic and betahistine medications and to continue to work on reducing my sodium intake. In addition, I should be working to avoid fluctuations in my sodium, making sure to avoid sudden spikes in my sodium consumption such as might occur by eating a high-sodium food item.

Although I thought I had been doing pretty well at reducing my sodium over the past few months, our conversation revealed how poor of a job I had actually been doing. I was eliminating the blatant sources of sodium but still consuming high amounts due to things like injected meats, canned vegetables, or bottled salad dressing. It was going to need to be a lifestyle change, and given the progress I had made while doing a relatively poor job of reducing my sodium previously, I was reinvigorated and ready to take the challenge head-on. If I didn't commit to the low-sodium lifestyle or, even worse – if it didn't work – we would have to look into the next stage of treatments, including steroid injections. I wasn't yet ready for needles being stuck into my ear.

To say that I threw myself into reducing sodium would be an understatement. Unfortunately, I didn't see the return to normalcy as quickly as I had after I first tried the sodium reduction. Three weeks later, my daughter was born. I remember holding her, still feeling the effects – albeit somewhat diminished – and being angry that this moment that everyone talks about, when you first hold your daughter, is being robbed by the constant anxiety brought about by Ménière's. Though I was thrilled, excited, and every other joyful feeling that comes with a newborn, those feelings were again suppressed as a result of the Ménière's symptoms. No more attacks had arrived, but I experienced enough lingering symptoms that I felt only a guarded optimism towards continued improvement.

Over the next few weeks the symptoms continued to diminish. By the end of July, I felt as though I was back to normal. But to avoid any chance of my symptoms regressing back to where they had been, I became religious about monitoring the sodium content of what I ate. In doing so I soon regained a lease on life that I was not going to let slip me by.

Chapter 4
My Symptoms

EXPLAINING THE VARIOUS SYMPTOMS of Ménière's to a
non-Ménière's patient is like explaining weightlessness to
someone who has never left the surface of the earth. You
can certainly describe the numerous symptoms, to which the
listener will nod and state that they feel your pain, but they will
never truly understand what the symptoms are like. Even now,
being free of Ménière's attacks for over six years has lessened my
memory of the misery that accompanies the instant vertigo and
constant headaches. If I as a former sufferer can't even mentally
replicate the hell of a vertigo attack, there's no way I should expect
a healthy person to grasp the desolation of Ménière's. Besides, I
would always just prefer an ounce of compassion anyway.

A couple of people have lightheartedly joked that my
description of Ménière's pretty much makes it sound like being
drunk. To an extent, there were times that I would agree with that.
The issue I took is when those same people would respond with
"*Cool!*". No, not cool at all, in any sense of the word. Though I
could appreciate their intentions, I can also state wholeheartedly
that having Ménière's is in no way 'cool'. It is beyond miserable.
Yes, being drunk can be fun, but being drunk usually occurs on
your schedule, in a setting which you have control over. Imagine

experiencing the effects of being drunk while at work, or church, or driving, or watching your kids play. Everyday. I doubt that anyone honestly thinks that it is 'cool' to feel drunk at those times, but for a Ménière's sufferer, they have no choice.

Because of the range of symptoms involved with my Ménière's, I have outlined in this chapter an overview of many of the symptoms I had during my time suffering from Ménière's. As you will see, Ménière's is not a consistent set of symptoms lumped together like the cough, runny nose, and sore throat of a cold. Rather, it is a combination of both ongoing as well as randomly occurring events, along with the acute vertigo attacks. Some symptoms are tolerable, some are annoying, and some are overwhelming. Your own experiences may vary, and you may or may not feel a variation of some, all, or any of these symptoms.

Again, one thing must be made clear when it comes to symptoms – your experience with Ménière's is unique to you. The symptoms I outline below were unique to me; therefore if you experience any variation of these symptoms it is not indicative of your having or not having Ménière's. Only a thorough dialogue between you and your physician can make that determination.

Ongoing symptoms

Tinnitus (ringing in the ears)

At some point we've all had ringing in the ears. It may have been after a loud concert, when we were congested due to a cold, or perhaps after we were standing too close to some holiday-themed cannon when it was fired. Temporary ringing in the ears in association with those events is perfectly normal but is not the type associated with Ménière's. I first noticed a constant ringing in my right ear about four years prior to my first attack. Initially, it was extremely annoying. Being in a very quiet room made it nearly unbearable, so some form of white noise like a fan or radio became a necessity. My tinnitus has always been a high-pitched "hiss" of sorts (around the 7500Hz tone, if you'd like to listen to it online). Whether it was directly related to my Ménière's or not is debatable, but given that it started in the same ear affected by Ménière's (my left ear eventually started to ring as well), an association between the tinnitus and Ménière's is not out of the question.

Varying tones, ear pressure, and diminished hearing

Once my attacks commenced, the high-pitched tinnitus started to vary in tone. I began to notice that my right ear exhibited a sensation of pressure, effectively the same as what someone feels when their ear is congested due to illness. With the pressure came a variety of constant sounds that served to drown out the aforementioned ringing in my ear. The sounds would range from a low hum to a loud, constant tone similar to the high pitch you used to hear on TV when those test-pattern color bars filled the screen, to a "whooshing" sound representative of something between the wind blowing through a tree and the sound of the crowd at a televised football game. The sounds and pressure were constant to some degree, save for a few rare days a year where they would disappear seemingly without reason (I later found that they disappeared for good when I went low-sodium, suggesting that these random fluctuations were due to temporary decreases in my dietary sodium).

A reduction in hearing along with a sort of 'pressure' in the ear are both common symptoms with Ménière's. For me, the ability to hear through my right ear was diminished tremendously. In hindsight, because my hearing has since returned to normal in my right ear (except for the continued high-pitched tinnitus), I feel that my previous issue of diminished hearing was more a result of the ear pressure "interfering with" my hearing than any actual damage resulting from Ménière's. When the ear pressure was present, I often had to turn and listen through my left ear as my right ear was relatively useless. Background sounds made conversation difficult, so any social gatherings for me involved honing in on key words and focusing on lip reading to try and piece together what was being said. This brought on quite a bit of anxiety for me. If someone said something to me from another room I somewhat feared the repercussions of my yelling "*WHAT?*" every time, especially because I suspected that they knew I was within earshot. Most of the time I would get up and walk to where the person was before apologetically asking "sorry, what did you say?".

Two more prevalent ear issues occurred with my right ear once the attacks started. The first is that sounds were both more metallic-sounding (some describe as "tinny"), which resulted in sounds being perceived as though they were occurring through a metal tube of sorts. This wasn't problematic necessarily, just annoying.

The second issue, however, was frustrating. Loud sounds were amplified, to the point that they would sometimes actually hurt. For example, I remember rummaging through pots in a counter one time. The sudden banging sounds of the pots hitting together were too much to take and I had to stop. Another time, ice from the dispenser falling into an insulated plastic cup hit just the right tone to make me pull away. A suddenly loud television commercial would be almost unbearable. Particularly frustrating was the fact that sounds were amplified despite the fact that my hearing was significantly diminished.

Nystagmus

Nystagmus is a condition of the eyes in which small, uncontrolled movements occur. To experience this sensation yourself, look at the header word "Nystagmus" above. Now, as fast as you can, shoot your eyes back and forth between the first and the last letters. You'll probably notice that your eyes fatigue pretty quickly and soon you're unable to continue. With true nystagmus however, this movement is uncontrollable and fatigue does not set in. In other words, the effects are constant. Every morning when I woke up the first thing I would do was open my eyes and stare at a spot on the wall. This was my own test of whether my symptoms were there. And every morning, the invisible spot on the wall would jump around uncontrollably.

I also found that if I tried to stare at a very small spot, such as a letter on a printed page, a unique event would happen. As I stared motionless for three or four seconds, I could feel a sort of tension building up inside my head. At the point it released, my eyes would shoot off to the side and then return back to where I had been staring. This wasn't necessarily problematic, unless I was focusing on a tiny object or attempting to read extremely small print such as the battery size stamped on the back of one of my watches. Over time, I found that I could avoid noticing the nystagmus if I randomly moved my eyes about. So instead of staring at a picture, I would move my eyes around to various spots on the picture. Focusing on a particular point is what made the nystagmus noticeable. Reading, driving, or normal life were tolerable as my eyes were able to move around constantly.

Pulling

One of the more strange sensations I felt was a 'pulling' sensation that would happen randomly. To understand this, imagine standing still and then being pulled to one side. That feeling you get *while you are in the process of moving* is the sensation I experienced. In other words, it's not the actual pull you would feel; rather, it's the sensation as inertia carries you through the movement. This would often occur while I was sitting still, which was particularly frustrating as it would cause me to physically move in response to the sensation. I could usually 'cover up' the sudden, random movement by acting as though I were simply shifting in my seat. Interestingly, ceasing my caffeine intake effectively stopped these pulling events from occurring – the only symptom of my Ménière's that I directly associated with caffeine. In the years since having stopped caffeine, even though I feel a random Ménière's symptom every now and then, I have yet to again have any pulling sensations.

Dizziness

We've all been dizzy before. For the healthy among us, any dizziness is typically due to issues such as spinning around or standing up too fast. In most cases, the dizziness is gone in a few seconds. My Ménière's-related dizziness was different. It felt just like the lingering sensation that you feel immediately after you stop spinning around. Not the spinning itself (that is the vertigo, which we'll get to later) but rather the after-effects. I was constantly dizzy to varying degrees. So much that when I turned my head rapidly I would often find myself squinting due to the uneasiness that the movement caused. Turning a corner while walking would sometimes bring on a brief but more intense bout of dizziness, which would soon subside. Though always present, the dizziness was tolerable and never caused any significant problem.

Unsteadiness

While the dizziness was annoying, the unsteadiness could be dangerous. The way I would describe my unsteadiness is to say that there were times that I felt as if the feedback to and from my legs was disconnected from my brain. Any unexpected change in the walking surface induced an imbalance issue for me. Similarly, an unanticipated, even microscopic amount, of tilting my chair would send a chill down my spine as I would get the sensation that I was falling. Chairs with a slightly loose seat that caused any kind of rocking motion were particularly problematic. Long hallways were troublesome as they could induce a sort of low-level vertigo that made it difficult to walk in a straight line, giving me a drunken sort of gait. The unsteadiness was not constant like the ear issues or the dizziness. Rather, it might be present for a week, or it might arise after a change in the walking surface. The dizziness was never severe enough to interfere with daily life or halt any of my outdoor runs, but it could cause a bit of anxiety at times.

Headaches

There was a time back when my symptoms first started that I had some form of a headache at all times. The headaches would fluctuate on a scale from about a 2 (very light) to about a 6 or 7 (moderate) at various points of the day, with no real indicator of what would improve or worsen the pain. Over time, the 'constant' headache dissipated. It was replaced with a new, more specific headache that would arise every few days in response to some event that my brain interpreted – incorrectly – as a loss in balance.

For example, one time I opened a set of interior double doors by pushing them forward. The rush of air that accompanied the opening of the doors actually pulled me through the door slightly, causing my brain to interpret this as my starting to fall forward. Within seconds, I had a headache for the rest of the day that felt like a large band across my forehead. Another time, I was walking on a sloping sidewalk (problematic enough on its own) when a small, unexpected gust of wind hit me from the side and caused me to momentarily lose my balance. That triggered a headache for the next few hours.

Additional headaches would arrive in various shapes and sizes, and they were impossible to predict. Fortunately they were manageable, and in my opinion never reached the degree of what I would classify as a 'migraine' based on stories I had read about migraine severity. Rather, they were uncomfortable at most, sometimes worsening as I leaned down or turned too fast. Since having gone on a low-sodium diet the headaches have for the most part disappeared.

Anxiety

The thought of an impending vertigo attack terrified me. It was on my mind constantly. Because of the ever-present variety of symptoms I would experience, it was hard to feel like an attack *wasn't* about to happen. This gave me two unique anxiety events. The first anxiety cause was due to the random fluctuation in symptoms – such as a sudden increase in dizziness – that made me feel as though an attack were imminent. This type of 'anxiety attack' would immediately increase my heart rate along with increasing the force of my heartbeat. I would instantly feel 'jittery'. Perspiration would begin. And I would frantically look around to develop an escape plan in the event that a full attack hit. All of these events would occur in a matter of 3-4 seconds, and given the variety of fluctuating symptoms the series of events may happen five or six or ten times a day. In effect, I was having multiple panic attacks per day.

The second type of anxiety I experienced centered around any particular scheduled event that I was responsible for. If I was required to be somewhere at a particular time my anxiety level would increase proportional to the closeness of the event. And you might be surprised when you really think about just how often your presence is *required* to be somewhere. If, for example, I had a meeting that required my attendance, I would be more perceptive of certain Ménière's symptoms as the meeting approached. Any small dizziness or imbalance event would be perceived as an impending attack. The anxiety arose from my fear that an attack would hit and I would miss the meeting, or the airport pickup, or the date, or the start of the experiment, which would in my mind turn into sheer chaos, annoyance, and misunderstanding for whomever else was involved. This constant concern served to make me perpetually anxious, with the exception of those few weekend days where I had no real outside responsibilities and could stay within the confines of my own schedule.

I had spoken to my physician about these events prior to my diagnosis with Ménière's and was prescribed alprazolam to counter the anxiety-related effects, but the drug had no effect and as a result I soon quit taking the medication. However, once on a low sodium diet the anxiety symptoms faded proportionally with my Ménière's symptoms.

Symptoms associated with Ménière's attacks

Vertigo

Of all my symptoms, vertigo was the worst. I absolutely feared the vertigo. The ear fullness, dizziness, unsteadiness, and related symptoms were tolerable. The vertigo was not. I tried many times to power through the vertigo attacks, but nothing I did would allow me to function normally once an attack hit. Even when intermixed with other symptoms such as sweating, or nausea, I most clearly remember the misery brought about by the sensation of the room or bed spinning like a tilt-a-whirl, with no possible way to get off.

To imagine vertigo as I experienced it is difficult. You might think you can just close your eyes and roll around, but consciously rolling around is controlled by your brain, so the brain automatically "accepts" the movement. You might try sitting in a chair, then have someone behind you place their hands on each side of your head and rapidly – 10 times – shake your head back and forth as if you are indicating "no". Then, imagine that same sensation only without the actual head movement. One event that replicated the sensation of my vertigo happened once while moving a giant mirror a couple years after my diagnosis. As someone moved the mirror unexpectedly while I was standing directly in front of it, I felt as though my surroundings shifted rapidly. It was intense and frightening enough (as a former Ménière's sufferer) that I had to step outside to regain my composure, given the memory of my intense vertigo attacks now again racing through my mind. Similar to the effects of the mirror, with vertigo you are not moving around but the brain perceives that you are. Closing your eyes does nothing, as you still feel as though the bed you are lying on is spinning in circles. There is literally no escape.

I also remember at least two visual effects from the vertigo. The first I would call "floating", in which the objects around me seemed to float around aimlessly. Imagine, almost, the sensation of looking around a room if there was no gravity. The objects around you would slowly be floating around at various speeds. That is how my vision would appear during some stages of vertigo. The effect was due to the involuntary motion of my eyes, but because my vision worked normally it appeared to me as though things were floating around the room. The second visual effect was more instantaneous and happened during the more severe vertigo attacks. I called the effect the "bowtie" response. During that kind of attack, the peripheral area of my vision would rapidly shake up and down, while the center of my view remained almost still. Viewed from my perspective, my field of vision resembled a giant bowtie of sort. Strange, indeed. But like Ménière's itself, it can be difficult to understand many of the individual effects.

The perfunctory effort

It's difficult to think of a word that captures the essence of "giving minimal effort", but *perfunctory* represents what having a Ménière's attack would relegate me to do. When the attack was occurring, I felt best if I could lay perfectly still with my eyes closed. I could still 'feel' the vertigo since the bed felt as though it were spinning – but I wanted to put forth no effort for anything. Even a sudden house fire might not have gotten me off of the bed. If I did perform voluntary exertion, it was always while using minimal effort. For example, if my car keys were in my pocket and making me uncomfortable enough to remove them, I would with a limp arm toss them over the end of the bed, letting my arm fall where it did and likely remaining there for the duration of the attack. Putting any unnecessary effort would cause my body to move, thereby increasing the misery of the vertigo. Phone calls would go unanswered, tasks would go unfinished. Because of the need to lie down, one technique I would often use if an attack hit at an inopportune time was to 'cancel' whatever I was working on. If cooking, I would quickly shut off the stove and make my way to a bedroom. If visiting someone, I would apologize quickly but rush to my car. To best manage the attacks, I needed solitude in order to remain as still and uninvolved as possible.

Profuse perspiration

Imagine lying still on a bed and perspiring a detailed outline of your body onto the bed. That is exactly what would happen to me during a full Ménière's attack. The sweat was profuse – occurring everywhere on my body – and rapid.

Several times I had a short bout of Ménière's symptoms that did not bring on a full attack but did induce enough anxiety to initiate perspiration. Rather than being perfuse in nature, these events brought on more of a 'cold sweat' in which I could feel the sweat on my skin but did not see it literally dripping off of my skin like I did during the major attacks.

Because I had two types of perspiration events I would often judge whether I was experiencing an impending full attack or not based on the type of perspiration that occurred. My Ménière's attacks weren't always "instant", meaning they didn't all induce sudden vertigo, nausea, etc., (remember the attack I described while sitting at the stoplight). If the perspiration increased or started to bead up on my skin I knew to suspect that a full attack was in progress. Other times, I would get hit with a bout of slight vertigo or increased unsteadiness that would start me perspiring, but the sweat remained very light on my skin such that I knew the symptoms would soon pass.

Nausea and vomiting

The final arrival to any Ménière's attack was the nausea, followed soon after by the vomiting. No matter how hard I tried to remain calm and quiet during the vertigo – with the hope of holding off the nausea event – I always ended up with a few minutes of nausea before a rapid onset of vomiting.

As I outlined in an earlier chapter, the vomiting was incredibly forceful. It didn't matter if there was something in my stomach or not – my body was going to clean it out regardless. Each retch would last four to five seconds, sometimes followed so closely by another that I could not even inhale. What struck me the most was the force by which so many of my torso muscles were involved. Every time I had a full attack, my upper shoulder muscles as well as a few in my neck felt the effects of the vomiting for the next couple of days.

Sleep

As the attack started to fade, the onset of a need to sleep became overwhelming. I called this time of the attack my "Ménière's nap". On the one side, I would welcome sleep because it meant the beginning of the end of the attack, in addition to an escape from any vertigo still present. On the other hand, once the attack was over I wanted to get up and go about my business, but sleep would delay that. Because the urge to sleep was so overwhelming it was simpler to not fight the urge and instead succumb to the two- to three-hour nap.

Post-attack symptoms

Hazy vision

Post-attack events were tolerable, mostly because I knew that they were temporary, only lasting for 24 hours or so after an attack. Starting as soon as I would wake up from the nap, everything I looked at seemed to have a haze, or inherent brightness. Being in a bright room or outside on a sunny day worsened the effect, and sunglasses were pretty much a requirement outdoors. Still, the haze had little effect on daily life and was more annoying than anything. By the next day, it would always be gone.

Brain fog

Although the haze was tolerable, the brain fog present for 24 hours or so after an attack was frustrating. After my first attack, the brain fog that I felt made me think that I had just experienced a seizure given that I had difficulty performing simple math on a calculator. Conversation, driving, or watching television was not a problem – it was "thinking" that took a slightly extended period of time, or in some cases took a lot more effort. Being a student at the time of my attacks, I did my best to avoid reading, calculating, collecting data, or typing out documents for a day or so after my attack because I knew that I could not trust the results. Thankfully, within 24 hours of an attack, the brain fog had always subsided.

The indescribables

The list of symptoms outlined above is not all-inclusive, but they capture the predominant symptoms present in some form during my symptomatic Ménière's period. You may experience the same, more, or other symptoms on your own. There were many more symptoms that occurred but were not consistent from day to day or – in some cases – defied description. It is difficult for a non-Ménière's sufferer to understand what a constant buzzing sensation, or a 'shock' sensation inside your head similar to the effect of touching an electric fence, or bubbling tingliness inside your skull, or rocks rolling down the back of your brain actually feels like. Yet that is how I often perceived many incidental symptoms.

As I stated earlier, it is difficult to explain Ménière's to someone who has not had it, probably much like it's difficult to explain the pain and feelings of childbirth to someone who has never gone through it. But nothing about Ménière's was painful for me. Rather, I felt overpowering sensations – dizziness, a disconnect with my limbs, vertigo, nausea, etc. None of those 'hurt' in the true sense of the word, but they are extremely debilitating all the same.

Because of the severity of some symptoms, it takes patience to understand what someone is going through when they have Ménière's. With the exception of excessive perspiration and perhaps seeing a Ménière's patient's eyes move with nystagmus, it is essentially impossible to feel what a Ménière's patient is feeling any more than a man can sense what a woman feels during labor and delivery. There has to be a level of compassion, which can often be all that a Ménière's patient asks for.

Chapter 5
The Role of Sodium

NEWLY DIAGNOSED MÉNIÈRE'S PATIENTS are often instructed to reduce their sodium intake. Because many Ménière's patients report an improvement in their symptoms after switching to a low-sodium diet, this chapter was designed to provide an overview of what sodium is, its function in our body, and how we interact with sodium on a daily basis. Understanding the intricacies of sodium can provide Ménière's patients insight into how sodium may influence the symptoms of Ménière's. In particular, outlining how we interact with sodium daily can help them become more cognizant of the sodium in their food, in turn providing them the means by which to make healthier food decisions.

Sodium as an element

Sodium is found in abundance within the earth's crust as well as its oceans. In its elemental form, sodium is highly unstable and reacts violently with oxygen and even water. Consequently, pure sodium is not found naturally in nature. Rather, sodium is found combined with a variety of other elements to form what is known as a compound such as sodium chloride (i.e. "salt") or sodium bicarbonate. The formation of a sodium-based compound alters the elemental structure of sodium, in turn transforming sodium from an atom into an *ion*. Once in its ion form, sodium becomes quite stable and can be used to perform its many tasks. Furthermore, the transformation of sodium into an ion supplies it with an overall positive electrical charge. It is this small but significant charge that provides sodium the power it needs to perform its vast array of functions.

Sodium's role in the body

Living organisms capture the power of the sodium ion in a couple of important yet very different ways. For example, our brains send nerve signals throughout our body by manipulating the position of sodium ions. Separately, sodium has a major role in regulating our body's fluid levels such that improper sodium levels can cause our bodies to either dehydrate or swell excessively. Detailing these processes below will hopefully give you both a better appreciation of sodium and help you understand why adequate sodium intake is vital for maintaining normal body functions.

Regulation of signaling

In order for many of our cells to function properly, sodium concentrations in and around the cell must be maintained precisely. When the cell is inactive, its internal sodium levels are low. The fluid surrounding the cell, however, maintains a high sodium ion concentration. Because of the positive charge each sodium ion holds, these unique sodium concentrations generate a unique electrical charge in each cell. Outside of the cell, the high concentration of sodium forms an overall positive charge. Inside of the cell, where there is little sodium along with many negatively-charged particles, a negative charge exists. When this balance of charges inside and outside of the cell is maintained – such as when the cell is at rest – it is called the cell's *resting potential.* When the brain initiates a command such as for a muscle to contract, cells transmit this command by manipulating their sodium concentrations, in turn altering each cell's resting potential.

In order to produce movement, our muscles require a signal from the brain, and sodium is highly involved in transmission of this signal. Once initiated by the brain, the signal is sent down a nerve through a series of events that manipulate the electrical charge in specific areas of the nerve cell's membrane. This occurs by reversing the internal and external cellular concentrations of the sodium ion along the nerve itself. To accomplish this change in the sodium concentrations, small sodium *channels* open on the cell membrane that allow sodium ions to rush into the nerve cell in one small area of the membrane. This rush of positively charged sodium ions, along with a series of other events, causes that area of the cell to become positive on the inside of the membrane and negative on the outside – effectively reversing the charge that exists when the cell is at rest – in a process called *depolarization.* This process of depolarization along a membrane generates what is called an *action potential.*

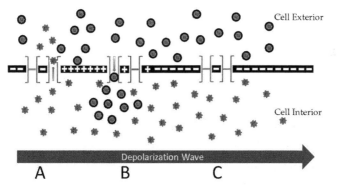

Figure 5.1. As sodium (shown as circles) enters the cell interior (B), the resting membrane potential changes polarity from negative (-) as in area A to positive (+) in response to the changing ion concentrations. Area C will eventually begin to change polarity in response to the changing membrane polarity in area B. Area A has already reverted back to (-) as the sodium has been removed from the cell interior

As one area of the cell membrane becomes depolarized it also depolarizes the area next to it (Area "B" of Figure 5.1). Simultaneously, the area that had just depolarized *(*Area "A" of Figure 5.1) begins to immediately remove the sodium ions from the cell interior using sodium *pumps.* As enough sodium gets removed, the membrane's resting potential is restored to resting levels while the action potential continues to spread along the nerve, eventually reaching the tissue of interest – such as a muscle – where the entire process eventually generates a muscle contraction.

The process of depolarization takes just milliseconds, and you might have yourself marveled at the speed with which it occurs had you ever reflexively jerked your arm back after touching a hot surface unexpectedly. Many processes within the body occur by way of nerve signal transmission, and it is clear that sodium plays a crucial role.

Regulation of fluid levels

The second major role of sodium in the body is to aid in the regulation of fluid levels. As discussed above, the body maintains a particular concentration of sodium ions both inside and outside of a cell. The body regulates these sodium ions in part via the bloodstream as well as through the kidneys. Decreased sodium within the body's tissues will trigger movement sodium from the bloodstream to the tissue area needed. Conversely, if the body's sodium levels are normal or begin to rise, the kidneys will filter sodium out of the blood and send the excess sodium out in the urine.

Strict regulation of sodium in the body is crucial. If tissue sodium levels become too high, the higher sodium concentration can actually pull water out of cells, creating a potentially deadly dehydration situation. Conversely, sodium levels that are too low can cause cells to swell in an attempt to remove water from the surrounding tissue. The science of how all of this happens is beyond the scope of this book, but makes for fascinating reading as it outlines how important of a role sodium has in the regulation of body fluids.

Clearly, maintaining proper sodium levels within the body is important for overall health. For Ménière's patients, however, it is even more important as failure to regulate sodium levels can have negative consequences for their Ménière's-related symptoms. As far back as 1934, Furstenberg showed an association between Ménière's disease and sodium retention, and was the first to recommend a reduction in sodium intake[26]. Since then, sodium restriction is commonly recommended as an initial treatment option by medical professionals, with moderate rates of success.

The main premise linking sodium with Ménière's centers around fluid maintenance within the inner ear. With Ménière's, it is largely thought that regulation of fluid within the ear becomes difficult to maintain due to a diminished capacity to regulate sodium levels. As we discussed earlier, without precise control of sodium concentrations, fluid levels can fluctuate. Whereas the sensitive inner ear consists of several membrane-encased fluids, any unregulated change in fluid levels can be problematic specific to pressure and/or potential rupture of the membranes. As such, it is theorized that maintaining a constant sodium level – rather than random peaks and valleys – can be beneficial to the Ménière's patient as it requires less effort to regulate sodium[21]. In addition, pharmaceutical aids such as diuretics can be used to help remove sodium from the body.

Sodium in the food industry

As discussed, sodium plays an extremely important role in the body. For sodium to perform its functions, there must be an adequate supply of sodium for the body to use. As our bodies cannot make sodium, it must be supplied externally through the food and drink that makes up our diet. Unfortunately, many diets today contain foods high in sodium which in turn contributes to many of the health problems that we as a society face. To understand why sodium is so prevalent in our diet we need to look at the reasons that sodium is present in so much of the food we eat. This chapter provides a brief overview of how the food industry utilizes sodium, along with outlining the rationale for adding sodium to many of our food products.

Sodium chloride

The predominant use of sodium in the food industry is in the form of sodium chloride. While we know sodium chloride under its more familiar moniker of "table salt" (or simply "salt), it also has specific uses in the food industry. Sodium chloride is utilized for flavor enhancement, and you will often hear that an under-salted food tastes bland. If you're somewhat of a food connoisseur, you may have even heard of or experienced the many various types of salt, such as sea salt, kosher salt, Celtic sea salt, or the beautifully pink Himalayan salt. With the exception of a few mineral "impurities" – such as iron which gives Himalayan salt its pink color – it is important to understand that all salts are effectively the same in terms of sodium content.

Besides our own desire to sprinkle some salt on our food, the food industry utilizes salt as a flavoring aid as well. Look at almost any food seasoning packet or boxed dinner and you can expect to see the inclusion of sodium chloride. Particular food items such as snack foods, frozen dinners, and seasoned meats are known to contain a high amount of sodium chloride and Ménière's patients should consume these items with caution. However, many of these items can now be found in lower-sodium options that may better fit some Ménière's diets.

The food industry's second major use of sodium chloride is to act as a preservative. As an example, vegetables themselves contain little sodium yet the label of a canned vegetable reveals an exorbitant amount of sodium. Why? Because the addition of a salty brine helps prevent the growth of pathogens such as bacteria or mold within the container. This in turn extends the shelf life of canned vegetables up to four years or more. By extending the shelf life, food products can be available year-round and production costs are kept low by limiting spoilage. Other processes are available for food preservation such as using high temperatures during the canning process or a combination of multiple preservation techniques, but because of its effectiveness and low cost, the most effective procedures typically involve some form of sodium addition.

Sodium as an essential ingredient

While sodium chloride plays a major role in taste and in food preservation, certain sodium compounds play a role in the development of the food itself. The ingredient list of almost all baked goods will include either sodium chloride or sodium bicarbonate, as both play a key role in the structure of the food. Sodium chloride is often added to yeast-based breads as it helps strengthen the gluten structure of the bread. Sodium bicarbonate is found in baked goods such as cookies and brownies that don't utilize yeast but still require the formation of carbon dioxide to generate the bubbles that are essential for the food's texture. As the sodium bicarbonate reacts chemically with another recipe ingredient such as milk, carbon dioxide is produced. Without the generation of that carbon dioxide, the food would be flat and difficult to chew. Sodium bicarbonate supplies the sodium ions required to provide an 'airiness' to the food product.

Besides the food industry, sodium is also prominent within the pharmaceutical industry. For example, sodium bicarbonate is an effective stomach acid neutralizer and is therefore found in high amounts in effervescent antacid tablets. As an example, the "Drug

Facts" label from the back of a common effervescent antacid label lists the sodium bicarbonate content as "(heat treated) 1916mg" *per tablet*. Furthermore, the recommended dosing schedule is two tablets every four hours, which provides an extreme amount of sodium in a very short time frame. Other common over-the-counter drugs such as naproxen sodium also contain inherent sodium, albeit in a much lower amount (e.g. 20mg per capsule) than antacids.

Summary

Given the prevalence of both processed foods and baked goods, it is no surprise that Americans consume on average 3,400mg of sodium a day. This is much higher than the recommended intake of 2,300mg per day, yet far exceed the body's actual requirement of sodium which has been suggested to reside around 500mg per day. Ménière's patients already on a sodium-restricted diet should be diligent in monitoring the sodium quantity of all food and drink consumed, including individual recipe ingredients. Doing so will help ensure that sodium levels remain steady and within a range that can help diminish some of the problematic symptoms associated with Ménière's.

Chapter 6
My Sodium Solution

PRIOR TO MY DIAGNOSIS with Ménière's I had two nutritional vices in life. They weren't typical vices such as overeating, or having too much junk food. Rather, my weaknesses were based around those little things that you don't need but you really want to have sometimes. For one, I enjoyed more than my fair share of salt. I added salt to seemingly everything: meats, vegetables, soups, whatever. I ate high-sodium snacks like seasoned crackers and microwave popcorn, often adding my own salt 'just because'. Even as a kid I remember thinking that a hearty Midwestern meal of meat and potatoes just didn't look right without the shimmer of a nice coating of salt. Whereas I was active, healthy, and even had great blood pressure I had no inclination to reduce my sodium intake.

My second vice was caffeine. I had never been a morning person, so once college life arrived I developed a habit of enjoying around ten or so cups of coffee per day, mostly before 9am. Within a few hours of finishing the coffee you could expect that I would down a caffeinated soft drink or two as well. As long as I cut the caffeine out by 6pm or so, I had no issues sleeping. Much like my attitude towards sodium, I saw no reason to consider cutting back on my caffeine as it helped me get going in the morning and didn't keep me up at night. In fact, I adapted so much to these vices that at one point I jokingly told a friend that I only plan on disobeying a doctor's orders twice – when he or she tells me to 1) stop drinking caffeine, or 2) cut down on my sodium.

Hindsight now reveals just how powerful my Ménière's symptoms must have been, given that I quit cold-turkey both my sodium and caffeine use within months of each other in 2011. Were Ménière's only causing infrequent pain or perhaps a light headache every now and then, I almost certainly would have continued using both sodium and caffeine without concern. Instead, because of the relief of my Ménière's symptoms I have remained caffeine-free and have not once added sodium to my diet for more than six years.

Things to consider . . .

Since my diagnosis in 2011, the improvement in health that I experienced after cutting my sodium intake turned me into a somewhat fanatical low-sodium enthusiast. I became passionate about the sodium content of my food and dove into learning an array of techniques designed to help maintain a low-sodium lifestyle. This chapter is designed to outline for you those tips and tricks that have helped me be successful in reducing my sodium intake to a level that still allows me to maintain an active yet Ménière's-free lifestyle.

As we will discuss, the techniques I outline in this chapter have been successful at nearly eliminating my Ménière's symptoms. Understand though, that Ménière's is not a one-size-fits-all condition; rather, everyone experiences their own symptoms and finds their own best treatment. I infrequently have very mild flare-ups that serve to remind me that my Ménière's is still lurking in the background. However, those rare events have nowhere near the ferocity and debilitating effects that they did while I was consuming a traditional diet high in sodium. Although I have no definitive link proving the association between my switching to a low-sodium diet and the improvement in my symptoms, the timing of the two events is highly convincing. And the fact that I have not had any additional Ménière's attacks while maintaining a low-sodium diet over the past six years lends further evidence that my Ménière's responds favorably to a low-sodium diet.

One final thought before we get into this chapter's content. As I said, the tips and techniques I lay out in this chapter were successful for me. They worked with my particular Ménière's condition and symptoms. And, these techniques were developed over time, by me, on my own. They were not hashed out around a conference table full of scientists and dieticians. Therefore, be clear about five important issues as you read through this chapter.

1) Understand that I am not a physician. I am a Ménière's patient who had success in reducing his symptoms through the reduction of my daily sodium intake. Therefore, none of the tips or techniques in this chapter should be considered medical advice. Rather, they serve to outline what worked and still works for me. Should you choose to enter into a similar low-sodium lifestyle after consulting with your physician, you may or may not have similar, worse, or better results.

2) If you think that changing to a low-sodium lifestyle can help your Ménière's, discuss the idea along with all of your available options with your physician before you begin. Only you and your physician can decide if a low-sodium lifestyle is best for you. Get a physical if your physician recommends one so as to ensure that your body is ready to take on a low-sodium lifestyle.

3) If you decide to reduce your sodium intake, do not jump full-speed into the techniques outlined in this chapter. Rather, make a slow and steady transition into a low-sodium diet so that your body is able to adapt to the reduction in sodium intake, something that it may not have experienced at any point prior.

4) Pay attention to what your body is telling you. If you feel 'strange', exhibit weakness, have no energy, or develop changes in

your Ménière's situation after transitioning to a low-sodium lifestyle, stop what you are doing and discuss those issues with your physician. Your body is designed to be healthy; any negative symptoms associated with entering a low-sodium lifestyle are likely indicative of an underlying problem, so discuss what you are feeling with your physician. Your Ménière's likely makes you feel miserable already. Treatments such as a low-sodium diet should make you feel better, not worse.

5) Understand that reducing your sodium intake needs to be a lifestyle change, not a quick fix. Therefore, make sure you have the right mentality before transitioning towards a lower-sodium diet. For example, are you willing to refrain from fast food? Restaurant food? The amount of sodium in fast food is extreme, often exceeding 1,000mg for one main menu item. To outline just how problematic sodium can be at fast food locations, look at the values below. Each category represents the sodium range (in milligrams) of a main menu item, taken across five fast-food restaurants for each item:

* Hamburger: 836-1372mg
* Large Pizza (two slices): 588-817mg
* 6" Sandwich: 1101-1203mg
* Beef/Steak burrito: 1270-2210mg

If your mindset is anything less than 100% for taking on a low-sodium diet, you'll likely become frustrated soon after starting. This can lead to difficulty adhering to the lifestyle, which can be problematic for a Ménière's patient given how fluctuations in sodium levels can trigger Ménière's symptoms. So if you aren't sure as to whether a sodium lifestyle is for you, wait until you have the right attitude to see the lifestyle through to fruition before committing.

Learning the basics, setting my standards

My official entry into a low-sodium lifestyle came about in the months after my final, most severe attack. It was then that I began to focus on making legitimate sodium-based changes to my diet. After my initial diagnosis I had made some changes, but I didn't understand at the time the true reach of sodium within the food industry. Instead, I made 'generic' changes by eliminating well-known, high-sodium food options such as soups, fast food, barbecue, etc. I didn't realize at the time that I was still consuming plenty of other foods without being aware of or even looking into the sodium level. During this phase – in between my diagnosis with Ménière's and my final severe attack, I had lingering symptoms but was nowhere near the level of miserable I had been for the previous three years.

After my final attack in May of 2012 I was frustrated, depressed, angry, and defeated all at once. A return trip to my neurotologist helped me understand that although I had cut out some sodium from my diet, I was still taking in a significant amount. So much, in fact, that even another drastic reduction in sodium would still leave me well within the acceptable range. As I started to research more into sodium and food, I realized the extent of sodium's reign. And I started to look deeper into physiology, both regarding how sodium worked as well as how much sodium was really required for a body to function normally.

What I quickly found was that there was a tremendous chasm of difference. Most Americans take in over 3500mg of sodium, yet the body only truly requires 500mg or so to function. However, 500mg should not be a daily, dietary target for multiple reasons. For one, the listed sodium content of food is derived from either a chemical analysis of the entire food item or by adding together the sodium contents of the individual ingredients. Even small errors in food consumption estimations could result in a much lower sodium intake than expected. For example, if the sodium content of a particular food item is based on an eight-ounce serving, and you consumed one spoonful – without weighing out the food, how confident are you that you had eight ounces of food? An estimation that you took in 100mg of sodium could easily end up actually being only 50mg, in turn reducing your overall sodium intake as well. Second, 500mg is assuming relatively sedentary activity. Any activity such as exercise would require a higher sodium intake due to increased sodium excretion. Therefore, 1000mg or 1500mg daily sodium intakes are typically recommended for Ménière's patients.

Using this information, one of the first things I did was to establish my sodium intake. I started off at 1500mg per day which was quite a challenge initially. However, the reduction in my Ménière's symptoms made the effort to cut excess sodium quite motivating. Going from constant anxiety and random four-hour bouts of vertigo to significantly reducing my Ménière's symptoms is a great motivator for doing what is necessary to ensure that the attacks don't return. Because my symptoms took a couple of months after my last attack to fully dissipate, I slowly progressed to a 1000mg daily intake of sodium around the time my symptoms largely disappeared. This in turn became my new daily sodium target.

The Nutrition Facts label

My biggest ally in the switch to a low-sodium diet was the Nutrition Facts label (Figure 6.1). This label – usually found on the back or side of a processed food package – outlines the particular food item's nutrient content per serving. Despite the label listing the major nutrients, I was focused squarely on the sodium content of the food. Because the Nutrition Facts label lists the sodium content *per serving* rather than 'per container' (near the top of the label), total sodium consumption must be calculated based on the amount of food eaten (i.e. serving size) *and* the sodium content per serving. For example, a can of no-salt-added green beans might list 20mg of sodium per serving. This does not mean that eating the whole can of green beans provides 20mg of sodium; rather, eating the entire can of green beans would supply 70mg of sodium as there are 3.5 servings per can.

Nutrition Facts	
Serving Size 1 cup (110g)	
Servings Per Container About 6	
Amount Per Serving	
Calories 250	Calories from Fat 30
	% Daily Value*
Total Fat 7g	**11%**
Saturated Fat 3g	**16%**
Trans Fat 0g	
Cholesterol 4mg	**2%**
Sodium 300mg	**13%**
Total Carbohydrate 30g	**10%**
Dietary Fiber 3g	**14%**
Sugars 2g	
Protein 5g	
Vitamin A	7%
Vitamin C	15%
Calcium	20%
Iron	32%

* Percent Daily Values are based on a 2,000 calorie diet. Your daily value may be higher or lower depending on your calorie needs.

	Calories:	2,000	2,500
Total Fat	Less than	55g	75g
Saturated Fat	Less than	10g	12g
Cholesterol	Less than	1,500mg	1,700mg
Total Carbohydrate		250mg	300mg
Dietary Fiber		22mg	31mg

Nutrition Facts	
6 servings per container	
Serving Size	1 cup (110g)
Amount per 1 cup	
Calories	**250**
% DV*	
11%	**Total Fat** 7g
16%	Saturated Fat 3g
	Trans Fat 0g
2%	**Cholesterol** 4mg
13%	**Sodium** 300mg
10%	**Total Carbs** 30g
14%	**Dietary Fiber** 3g
	Sugars 2g
	Added Sugars 0g
	Protein 5g
7%	Vitamin A 1mcg
15%	Vitamin C 2mcg
20%	Calcium 4mcg
32%	Iron 5mg

* Percent Daily Values are based on a 2,000 calorie diet. Your daily value may be higher or lower depending on your calorie needs.

	Calories:	2,000	2,500
Total Fat	Less than	55g	75g
Saturated Fat	Less than	10g	12g
Cholesterol	Less than	1,500mg	1,700mg
Total Carbohydrate		250mg	300mg
Dietary Fiber		22mg	31mg

Figure 6.1. A representation of the old (left) and new (right) Nutrition Facts label. Pay particular attention to the sodium content as well as the serving size and 'contents per serving' for an accurate representation of sodium

Serving size is important to understand as some items such as canned green beans will have multiple servings per container, while other items such as soft drinks, snacks, or carrots have serving sizes based on one package or item, such as one can of soft drink or one snack food item. Ménière's patients must be aware of this, as a misunderstanding could factor significantly into their overall sodium consumption. For example, some snack crackers come in a package of six, with 250mg of sodium per serving of three crackers. The small size of the package may lead a consumer to assume that one package is equal to one serving when in fact each package contains two servings. Such a simple miscalculation can quickly lead to significant variances in an individual's sodium intake.

Setting a budget and sticking to it

Analysis of the food nutrition label revealed to me that many of the foods I was still eating contained a sodium level much higher than what would be allowed for what I termed my "sodium budget", or the amount of sodium I allowed myself to consume per day. My sodium budget became my guide, in the same way a daily or monthly financial budget works. You may want a new TV or maybe even a nice pair of shoes, but the cost is more than your budget can handle. Likewise, if I craved a particular food item, say a fast food burrito, the 1,200mg of sodium used up my entire daily sodium budget in one item. Therefore, it was relatively easy to talk myself out of high-sodium foods that I may occasionally crave.

A lot of my sodium budget is planned in conjunction with a cost-benefit ratio for my diet. What that means is that if a food has very little satiety (i.e. hunger satisfying) value, such as a snack cake, it is not worth eating if the sodium content per serving reaches a value that I considered too high, usually around 130 to 140mg or more. In other words, eating a snack cake that has 140mg of sodium is a relatively high cost to my sodium budget with little benefit (i.e. not feeling full) in return. However, ¾ cup of popcorn kernels turns into quite a big bowl of popcorn. Using a little vegetable oil and seasoning with some salt substitute and a teaspoon of parmesan cheese provides less sodium overall but is a much larger, more filling snack, hence a much higher cost-benefit ratio. I have found that eating something small with little satiety value would increase my chance of continuing to 'graze', thereby increasing the likelihood of my consuming additional, unnecessary sodium.

This cost-benefit ratio applies to meals as well. For example, using low-sodium ingredients I could easily make a huge pasta salad for lunch, or a delicious Salisbury steak dinner, and end up completely full. A smaller store-bought version of those same two meals would supply 400% and 700% more sodium respectively for a smaller amount of food. By making the food myself I am able to get more food for much less overall sodium than if I purchased those same meals in a store.

To get this higher cost-benefit ratio, cooking my own low-sodium meals just made sense. It started after my final Ménière's attack when I finally recognized the high sodium content of the prepared foods my wife and I had been eating. I had for years been cooking for myself in order to save money as a student, but those meals were largely boxed dinners, frozen meat patties, or other prepared meals loaded with seasoning packets or canned sauces – all foods which I could no longer afford on my sodium budget.

The thought of prepping your own meals may put an unhealthy fear into some people, but given the extensive benefits, I can't recommend it enough for Ménière's sufferers. It saves money, makes you a more informed Ménière's patient, and perhaps most importantly it guarantees that you are in charge of the sodium content of your food. Dining out or eating food prepared by someone else always brings me a sort of edginess in that I cannot guarantee that the food was prepared to my low-sodium requirements. The first time I go to a new restaurant I can usually find their nutrition facts menu online, but these menus are problematic in and of themselves. I tend to be skeptical of much about these menus, as they only reflect the sodium value of the food item that was sent in for analysis. As such, a cook could easily alter the sodium content of the same menu item by adding a bit extra seasoning inadvertently. Therefore I tend to relegate myself to some carefully selected low-sodium sides or when possible I order the food unseasoned. Eating out is still feasible, it just takes a little extra work which we'll discuss later in this chapter.

Although I had the mindset for cooking all of our meals, time became one of the biggest barriers. Working ten hours a day as a post-doctoral associate at a medical college, along with my wife working as many or more hours at her job, and having an infant in the house, did not make coming home to another hour of meal preparation and cooking very inviting. There were many times I was tempted to throw together a few packs of microwaveable macaroni and cheese, or stop on the way home for a few burger-and-fry meals at a fast food joint. I began to understand why America's health was so bad – anyone pressed for time quickly realizes that the convenience of fast food is immensely easier than cooking a full meal. But I held the belief that the investment of my time involved in cooking was much more acceptable than the consequences of my Ménière's flaring up again. And every day that I felt normal was certain validation for the time I had spent on meal preparation.

Ingredients make the dish

I quickly found that there are a wealth of recipes available online that target low-sodium cooking. What I also found is that many of them fail to grasp the concept of "low-sodium" in that they call for ingredients with relatively high amounts of sodium and then simply throw in a salt substitute in place of regular salt. Personally, I fail to see how a 500mg or 680mg serving of a dish is exactly low-sodium, yet these values were often listed in recipes designated as low-sodium. I surmised that the recipe author assumed that this new recipe is *lower* sodium than the original which included salt instead of salt substitute. I soon learned that the key to a successful low-sodium diet is to start with sodium-friendly ingredients. For example, a can of regular diced tomatoes, with 3.5 servings per can at 280mg of sodium per serving – for a total of 980mg of sodium per can – could easily be replaced with a no-salt-added, identically sized can of diced tomatoes containing only 20mg of sodium per serving (i.e. 70mg per can). In other words, I could use one can of regular diced tomatoes and effectively meet my sodium budget for the day, or I can use a no-salt-added version and use less than 10% of my budget with no real sacrifice in flavor.

Over time, I began to find other low-sodium or no-salt-added versions of foods that are traditionally high in sodium. Canned vegetables. Un-injected meats. Snack crackers. Very-low sodium soy sauce. Packaged pizza crusts. These low-sodium options opened a wealth of new recipe options, and every new low-sodium item I found introduced even more recipes. Even most ingredients had some form of low-sodium or sodium-free sibling. Salt itself had a sodium-free substitute – potassium chloride – that could be used in place of salt (though some claim it has a distinct, noticeable taste). Baking powder, which rivals salt itself in terms of sodium content, comes available as a sodium-free version. And one Christmas, my wife surprised me with what may be my most appreciated gift ever – sodium-free chicken bouillon that I did not even know existed. I immediately was able to re-discover soups and various recipes that I'd had to avoid since my diagnosis given the high sodium content of bouillon.

In my search for low-sodium ingredients I learned that two identical-sounding products on a shelf can be vastly different in sodium content. For example, some brands of chili powder contain just that – sodium-free, 100% chili powder. Others, despite the identical label of 'chili powder', contain a variety of salt and other ingredients that can push the sodium content up over 150mg per teaspoon. Similarly, meats like chicken are naturally low in sodium, typically ranging from 45 to 80mg of sodium per serving. However, many processors inject some form of brine or add seasoning to their meat which can push the sodium content per serving up over 600mg or more. This difference in sodium content is why it is imperative that Ménière's patients check the Nutrition

Facts label and ingredient list of every item prior to purchase, as identical items of food (e.g. drumsticks) can have a ten-fold or higher difference in sodium between manufacturers.

It should be noted that while many foods and ingredients can be found in sodium-free versions, striving to use as many sodium-free ingredients as possible is not recommended. Remember that our bodies need sodium, and as a result consuming zero sodium over time in any diet is extremely dangerous and can be fatal. With the exception of perhaps fruits, some of which are extremely low in sodium, sodium-free items that I eat are always consumed with some other sodium-containing ingredient. For example, sodium-free tortilla chips are always eaten with salsa. Pasta is covered in meat sauce. Rice is topped with meats or vegetable mixes. Popcorn is mixed with a little grated parmesan cheese. Though my mindset is focused on maintaining a low-sodium diet, I am at the same time careful to design a diet that provides a healthy amount of sodium.

When low-sodium isn't an option

If a low-sodium food is not available, a little creativity still allows me to enjoy many foods. For example, certain ingredients such as lemon or lime juice can provide a hint of salt flavoring to meat, pasta, or rice dishes. Or, if perhaps I am away from home and the store only has traditional canned vegetables, I can easily rinse the vegetables in tap water to remove as much sodium brine as possible. I've also done this for seafood such as fish that are often coated with salt prior to freezing. Understand, though, that rinsing does not remove *all* sodium, as the long-term soak in a sodium brine has allowed the sodium to permeate into the food itself. One alternative I have used to help remove additional sodium is to soak the food in tap or even deionized water as well.

When rinsing or soaking is not feasible for removing sodium, I look into ingredient substitutions. For example, cheddar cheese isn't regularly available in a low-sodium option. However, Swiss cheese is naturally lower in sodium than most all other cheeses. So for a small but unique change in the recipe, I sometimes replace higher-sodium ingredients with ingredients containing significantly less sodium. In some cases, if I don't want to change the flavor of a recipe drastically enough to use a substitute, I simply reduce the amount of the high-sodium ingredient. My pizzas, for example, are made with a low-sodium crust, no-salt-added tomato sauce, Swiss cheese, ground beef, and sliced vegetables. But I still sprinkle on a little mozzarella for authentic pizza flavor despite its relatively high sodium content compared to Swiss.

Remember, too, that many foods naturally contain sodium. Meats, fish, and even many vegetables contain inherent amounts of sodium. For example, one carrot or one stalk of celery can provide from 50-70mg of sodium. A frozen, plain fish fillet can provide from 40-100mg of sodium. Therefore, with a healthy, balanced diet you can expect to consume much of your essential sodium just by eating healthy foods. Adding sodium at the dinner table for flavor is not generally needed, but may be permitted based on your own budget. For me, the desire for salty flavor was quickly outgrown. Instead, what was once a required taste in my food has now become somewhat of an alarm as I can quickly detect salty flavor, leading me to likely pass on consuming the remainder of the food item as I cannot be confident of its sodium content.

Develop your own recipe library

Eventually, understanding all of these low-sodium intricacies led to cooking becoming a passion, and I started looking for unique recipes. I soon learned that there were almost no recipes that I could not replicate and transform into a low-sodium version. My internet searches began including the words '*from scratch*'. I began to *exclude* certain results from my internet searches as well, such as "soup mix", which contributed a tremendous amount of sodium. I categorized certain types of recipes by preparation time, allowing me to quickly find the fastest recipes on the days I was shortest on time. And I began to develop a stockpile of recipes that were built around foods with low-sodium contents, such as ground beef, rice, or pasta. These complexities began to make cooking fun and a bit challenging, all the while knowing that not only was I keeping myself relatively Ménière's-free, but I was also providing healthy, home-cooked meals for my family.

Sample Recipe

To outline how a hearty recipe can still be low in sodium, I have detailed below one of my favorite recipes – spaghetti with meat sauce. This is one of the first recipes that I came up with and it is still a favorite in my family. As written, this entire recipe – not just one serving – provides just 245mg of sodium. In comparison, a half cup of most store-bought pasta *sauces* contains from 300-500mg of sodium or more. As you can see in this recipe example, simply utilizing low-sodium ingredients and excluding salt results in just a fraction of total sodium that a comparable recipe made from prepared ingredients (e.g. bottled sauce) would supply.

Ingredients (total sodium mg):
* *1/3 pound ground beef (110)*
* *1 tsp olive oil (0)*
* *½ yellow onion, diced (10)*
* *½ green pepper diced (5)*
* *1 can (14.5 oz), no-salt-added petite-diced tomatoes (50)*
* *1 can (8 oz) no-salt-added tomato sauce (70)*
* *½ tsp garlic powder (0)*
* *1 tbsp finely chopped basil (0)*
* *1 tsp oregano (0)*
* *½ tsp black pepper (0)*
* *16 oz spaghetti (0)*

Directions

In a skillet, sauté the onion and green pepper in the olive oil until soft (approximately 5 minutes). Remove from the pan and then brown the ground beef. Once brown, add the onions and peppers back in, along with the diced tomatoes, tomato sauce, garlic, basil, oregano, and black pepper and heat to a boil, then reducing to a simmer for ten minutes. While simmering, cook the spaghetti per package directions, and then drain. Plate a large helping of spaghetti and then add the meat sauce over the top.

Package labels

When looking at low-sodium foods and ingredients you will come across several different explanations of the item's sodium content, and it is important to be aware of the differences in label claims as they have the potential to be confusing. The Food and Drug Administration has established food labeling guidelines which outline what can and cannot be listed on a food label. And, there are restrictions as to how sodium content can be described.

Common labeling tactics you will see on food packaging include *sodium-free, no salt added, or lightly salted*, among others. Even though each label indicates a reduction in sodium, there can be significant differences in the sodium content. As outlined below, food package claims must meet specific sodium requirements in order for the manufacturer to make that claim[27].

Sodium Free, Salt-Free: *Less than 5mg of sodium per serving*
Very Low Sodium: *35mg of sodium or less per serving*
Low in Sodium: *140mg of sodium or less per serving*
Light in Sodium: *At least 50% less sodium than an original, comparable item*
Reduced/Less Sodium: *At least 25% less sodium than the original item*

No salt added, Unsalted:*No salt was added during processing*
Lightly Salted:*50% less sodium than the original food item*

It is important that as a consumer you are aware of these food labels and what each label designation represents. This can help avoid confusion, in turn reducing the possibility of inadvertently consuming excess sodium. Personally, I recommend that you pay much less attention to the package claim than to the Nutrition Facts label, as the Nutrition Facts label directly outlines the total sodium content.

Dining out

Eating in the home tends to provide me a layer of security regarding my sodium intake that I can't get at a restaurant. Because I cook the food myself I have no apprehensiveness about sodium content. Therefore when I'm at home I can eat as much as I'd like without worry about sodium. Dining out, however, can introduce a few complexities that typically require a bit more planning.

Dining out should not be a source of anxiety for a Ménière's patient, but it does require that you remain cognizant of your food choices. Over time I have established a sort of restaurant ranking based on their menu and accommodations to my diet. Those restaurants that I have no problem frequenting (i.e. code "green") are either ones that I have established low-sodium options for, or serve extensive fresh fruit or salad options. In fact, one of my personal favorite menu "items" is a buffet with an included salad bar, as I can eat my fill of fresh vegetables and salad without worry. Other times, I crave tortilla chips and salsa, to which I have learned that some restaurants do not salt their chips. Restaurants that serve fresh-made meat patties or unseasoned steaks are also on my top recommendation list.

My second-tier restaurants (code "yellow") are those that I will patronize but expect to find limited low-sodium options. If I can work those limited options into a meal, I have no problem eating there. Usually I do this by combining "sides" such as a house salad and baked potato. As long as I can eat enough food to become "full", I feel that it has been a worthwhile experience.

The final group of restaurants are those that I avoid (code "red"), where almost *everything* is prepared with sodium-based ingredients. These restaurants are the most difficult. Barbecue and seafood restaurants fall into this group because there is not much there to eat other than maybe a side of coleslaw. Sure, it's possible that one or two of these restaurants have a lower-sodium content in their sauce than others, but I'm not willing to experiment to find that out. Seafood restaurants are notorious for adding salt-based seasonings, and many wait staff have told me that their menu items are packaged in a salt brine. This is understandable, as fresh seafood has a short shelf life and the vast majority of customers are unconcerned with their sodium intake.

I have found that most dine-in restaurants are quite accommodating to any sodium requests. Special diets are nothing new to restaurants in this low-sugar, gluten-free society. Yet, an understanding of low-sodium hasn't yet reached the popularity of other 'special diet' options. For example, a popular chain restaurant claims on its website that it has options no matter the dietary request. It then outlines its special menu options for diets sensitive to *milk, soybean, vegan, vegetarian, sulphites,* and *wheat & gluten.* Low-sodium is nowhere to be found. I'm not sure if this is because there are no real options available, or if it's just that requests for low-sodium options simply don't happen enough. Regardless of the true reason, such menu accommodations outline my frustration with the food industry's heavy reliance sodium, in that there just aren't many options available for those of us sticking to a low-sodium diet.

A low-sodium request, though it may gain you a strange glance from a waiter every now and then, should be no different. I have found, though, that wait-staff can be somewhat oblivious to their own establishment's use of sodium. For example, I have been told by a waiter that "we don't salt our fries", only to find out upon receiving the order that the seasoning had been added prior to packaging. The same can hold true with burger patties, steaks, or vegetable sides, depending upon how they were stored prior to use (e.g. canned, packaged with salt, etc.). I simply ask that they check first, and if there is any uncertainty I'll order something else. The notion of inquiring into unsalted food applies at fast-food restaurants as well, as I've found that I can get unsalted fries at many establishments. Though pizza, hamburgers, or burritos are typically off my low-sodium menu, fries and other sides may be available at many fast-food restaurants depending on each restaurant's preparation.

Social events

One of the most perplexing times for someone on a low-sodium diet is when attending social events. Holidays are particularly tough as there is a wealth of food available, prepared by those closest to us. For me, I can't be sure of the sodium content of most of the available food so I choose (regretfully, most often) to avoid the food rather than take on the risk. This mindset largely stems from one Thanksgiving prior to my diagnosis where I had two relatively strong attacks in two days. It was those attacks that first started my thought process that there was something about what I was eating that triggered these strange and miserable events. However, at the time I did not suspect sodium as I had relatively little knowledge of its power. Since my diagnosis, my awareness of sodium makes me even more suspicious of foods I did not prepare myself. As such, I will tend to avoid any food in which I am not highly confident of the sodium content. This typically relegates my holiday food consumption to dishes my wife or I prepared (such as my standard spaghetti with meat sauce outlined earlier) or one of the various desserts that are typically low in sodium. Holidays are not the only challenge, mind you. Besides the occasional night out that requires a restaurant visit, birthday parties are typically filled with baked goods containing ample amounts of sodium bicarbonate and salt. There have been times that the food options aren't within my sodium means. Therefore, I employ my most drastic sodium defenses. In those cases I will most likely decline to attend, choose to meet the group later, or, as happens most often, I will eat prior to attending and then enjoy the company of others as they eat. It may seem awkward but other than a few honest inquiries as to why I wasn't eating, I have never had an issue. There are times in the Ménière's life that you have to be a little bit selfish. Staying in control of your diet is definitely one of those times.

Summary

Taking control of my sodium and caffeine intake has had the most definitive impact on improving my Ménière's symptoms. I can say without hesitation that sodium reduction has effectively eliminated my symptoms, save for a few random but relatively uneventful blips that arise every now and then. As I outlined in the beginning of this chapter, sodium and caffeine maintenance may or may not work for you. What I am certain about though is that if you and your physician feel that sodium and/or caffeine reduction could be an effective component of your Ménière's treatment plan, you must adopt the mindset of making it a lifestyle change. There will likely be cravings, frustrations, and inconveniences along the way, but the possibility of improving your Ménière's symptoms can make the effort well worth your while.

Chapter 7
Life After Diagnosis

THE SUMMER OF 2012 essentially became my awakening party of sorts. The previous months had seen me embark on my initial low-sodium effort in addition to starting diuretic and betahistine medication, with mildly favorable results. After my vicious attack in May of 2012 I stepped up not only my sodium restriction but also my understanding of sodium itself. As my symptoms improved I gained a new appreciation for how I was feeling, and was determined to do what I needed to do to keep the momentum going. Still, while keeping an open mind I maintained a guarded optimism knowing how strong my most recent attack had been after consuming the pot roast. For the most part, I was elated that I kept feeling better week after week, yet a small part of me tempered my enthusiasm so as to prevent too much of a letdown should another attack surface.

If anything, I rationalized to myself that what occurred with the pot roast was actually a good thing. I likened it to a basketball team losing a game right before the conference tournament. Had the team not lost – and thereby realized their vulnerability, perhaps they would enter the tournament with a bit of complacency and ultimately lose to a lesser team. The pot roast incident forced me to return to my neurotologist where I was able to refocus on sodium as a potential culprit. I doubled down on my sodium reduction and became more cognizant of what products contained hidden sodium. I read pages and pages of websites outlining sodium in food. I started to apply and modify tips and tricks I read about in order to apply it to my own habits. I learned about sodium requirements in the body along with how sodium is removed from the body. And the more I focused on controlling my sodium, the better I continued to feel.

By the end of the summer, I classified myself as 99% back to normal. There were still little 'blips' every now and then, but no major symptoms and certainly no attacks. The 1% of the time I would be reminded of Ménière's paled in comparison to the remaining time that I felt great. It gave me a new perspective on life, and it was amazing. I no longer worried about rolling around on the floor with my daughter, or swimming underwater, both activities which I feared immensely during the days surrounding my prior attack. And the more activities I tried, the more confidence I would gain after getting through the activity with no issues. I could now walk down spiral staircases without feeling dizzy, or drive over a steep bridge without setting off a minor anxiety attack.

Being able to remove myself from the Ménière's leash I had been living on allowed me to focus on improving all aspects of my health. I had been running short distances of three to four miles on my own for years. As my understanding of sodium grew, it brought me a deeper understanding of the science of perspiration. I became particularly interested in the sodium content of sweat, which gave me the realization to use exercise as a tool to help regulate my sodium. Perspiration became both a device for removing sodium and an insurance policy in the event that I felt I took in a little too much sodium. And the heat and humidity of southeast Texas provided ample opportunity to sweat.

Over time I developed the attitude that longer runs would make me sweat more, in turn eliminating a greater amount of sodium. Dining out became less of a worry as I would simply go for a run prior, thereby ensuring that a little inadvertent sodium at dinner would not affect me. And as my fitness began to improve more from the increased running, I began to run longer. My competitive side that had been dormant for years while suffering from Ménière's was recharged. I would set a goal of running 4.5 miles for each run that week. The next week it was 5 miles. The next week I would try to run the same distance faster. The success I was having as my symptoms continued to improve was countered only by a slight reduction in sleep, as I would have to wake up earlier in order to complete my runs before my wife or daughter woke up.

New goals, new accomplishments

Around this time, I started to think that it was time to find a new fitness goal. Never having been a runner during my earlier years, I had eventually worked my way up to a few 5K races in the years prior to my first attack. Entering races stopped after my Ménière's started for fear of an attack occurring during or just prior to a race. I felt that not racing at all was more logical than the inconvenience of an in-race or pre-race attack that would cause concern at the race and force me to forfeit my entry fees. Now, having less fear of an attack interfering with scheduled events, I felt it was time to re-evaluate my race opportunities.

The rational step would have been to re-enroll in a 5K or even push for a 10K; but instead I challenged myself to a half marathon. Years earlier, before I was aware of the Ménière's, I had told my wife (then girlfriend) that a marathon was on my bucket list, but I had never pulled the trigger in time before my attacks hit. Now, with my newfound enthusiasm towards running events again I started to reassess whether a marathon was possible. And with the motivation of being Ménière's-free I felt that anything was possible. But first I had to conquer a half marathon.

The cold late-February morning of the race brought out a heightened case of the jitters I feel in pretty much every competition I have competed in, ever. This morning though, I saw those jitters as one part a reminder of how far I had come and one other part a welcome back into the competitive running life once again. So this day I welcomed the nervousness with open arms, the same way I welcomed every morning now – a sharp contrast to the dread I had felt every morning I woke up with Ménière's.

The race started well, and I was feeling great about my pace, fitness, and chances of finishing. The excitement of participating in a race again was quite motivating, and all of the memories of the past five years rushed through my head as I remembered thinking that I would never be able to walk normally or be free of the constant anxiety. And here I was, running down a city street surrounded by a few thousand other runners who were each filling their minds by thinking about their own issues. I remembered thinking of that old phrase that someone always has it worse than you do. Looking around that day, I knew that after having been through years of Ménière's and now running symptom-free in a half marathon, *everybody* that day had it worse than I did.

The race continued on and eventually I settled into a pace that I felt I could maintain for the rest of the race. At one point I was handed a carbohydrate pack from a race crew member. While looking over the package I noticed "caffeine" on the ingredients list. That was all I needed to see – I wasn't going to risk it. I tossed it off to the side along hundreds of other empty ones.

Two miles later it happened. At mile 11, I was running along the side of the road when suddenly a "bang" occurred inside my head forceful enough that I remember it physically causing my head to jerk to the side. To this day I don't know what it was, nor has it ever happened again. I quickly jumped up onto the median. A bit of unsteadiness was now evident, but it seemed to be dissipating. With just two miles to go I was doubly motivated to continue on, both to finish the race and to get to the finish line in the event that my condition worsened. I pushed on, hanging by the side of the road just in case it became serious and caused me to trip or fall.

Eventually, I made it across the finish line, but my elation was suppressed by the hazy vision and dizziness I was experiencing. I could walk and function normally, but the old sensation of feeling like I had just stopped spinning had returned. A part of me felt glad that I had discarded the carbohydrate pack, or else I would have associated my dizziness with the caffeine. Rather, I knew that Ménière's was lurking silently in the background, begging me to give it a chance to surface. But I wasn't going to give it that opportunity.

Within an hour of crossing the finish line things had returned back to normal. I knew that it hadn't been an attack, and given my absence of symptoms over the previous months I eventually chalked it up as a fluke. I was confident enough that I ran another half-marathon soon after. I wanted to prove to myself that there wasn't some strange running threshold that would trigger my Ménière's symptoms.

That next half marathon was fine for the first nine miles, but soon afterwards I had a rapid and powerful dizzy spell right in the middle of the road. It was enough that I immediately slowed to a walk and crouched down to ensure I didn't fall over. Ironically it happened right in front of one of the race crew police officers, who began to walk over to me. As quickly as the dizziness appeared, it started to fade. I looked up and motioned to the officer that I was going to be OK. To prove it, I stood up and began to walk, soon returning to a jog and eventually finishing the race.

I didn't enter another race for eight months, finally signing up for my third half marathon in December. Maybe it was the cooler weather, maybe it was just pure luck, but finally I completed a race without a Ménière's incident. This accomplishment gave me a new-found boost of confidence, which further motivated me to train harder and see what I could achieve if I put forth the effort. Two months later, my fourth half marathon also resulted in no incidents, and perhaps even more importantly I had cut almost fifteen minutes off of my finish time. I was ready to move on.

Raising the bar

I had joined an early morning running group with individuals from our neighborhood, and we had become a somewhat close-knit group. We would run at 5am, and range anywhere from five to eight miles as a group. Secretly, the half marathon bug had worn off and I was anxious to take the next step by advancing to a full marathon. But at the same time I had a slight fear of failure. Therefore, I decided to attempt a marathon yet I approached the idea with subdued expectation given that I hadn't run farther than a half marathon. Ever. Furthermore, I had lingering suspicions that running distance or some other underlying issue had triggered the Ménière's events at my first two half marathons, and I knew that they had a small chance of happening again, even though the last had been a year ago.

Never mentioning it to my running group, I signed up for a relatively small marathon 100 miles away in a town I had lived and worked previously. I figured that if I failed to complete the marathon, no one would ever know, and I could at least get a nostalgic trip out of it. The morning of the mid-March race was unusually cold, and I quickly realized that I had underdressed. Yet, other than a flare-up of some minor hip pain that had been following me for a couple of weeks, the race was surprisingly uneventful and I finished just over four hours after starting. Most importantly, no Ménière's events. I was ecstatic two times over – I had completed a marathon and I was able to run 26.2 miles without a Ménière's attack.

Throughout the previous year, my Ménière's had been relatively held in check. I may have had a few days every now and then where I would have a few seconds of unsteadiness, but nothing of any concern. And never did I suspect that I was regressing back to the level of Ménière's from a few years earlier. With each passing day I became more and more convinced that my low sodium diet was the effective treatment I needed, and by no means was I going to risk any possibility of going back where I once was. I had even long ago stopped taking my medication – both the betahistine and the diuretic – and had no regrets. I felt that the combination of exercise and the low-sodium diet were effectively controlling my sodium, and the lack of significant symptoms from those two efforts alone had as much or more effect than the medication had provided.

Twice during my runs I had an incident that I attribute to my low-sodium intake. The first happened within days of reducing my sodium. While on a short three-mile run on a hot day in June, I felt an initially strange, warm sensation in my stomach area. As I continued, the sensation spread out across my body like a wave, bringing on a feeling of fatigue in my limbs that forced me to slow my gait to a walk. I also noticed that I had grown a bit 'jittery', with my hands making small, rapid movements similar to shivering. While relatively uneventful other than causing fatigue, it quickly passed and I was able to resume running without incident. This same event happened again at mile 18 of my second marathon. Two minutes later, I was back to my running pace. I don't know what exactly these events were, nor whether they were directly related to my low sodium intake. Given their extremely rare frequency (twice in five years of long-distance runs) along with the fact that they lasted no more than 3-4 minutes, I have not been too concerned about their occurrence. My belief is that if these events were in fact the result of my low sodium intake, the benefit of the reduction in Ménière's symptoms far outweighs the brief annoyance that they bring.

Water is no obstacle

In April of 2015, I volunteered along with some of my colleagues and students at a half-Ironman event 50 miles from home. Though my duty was to provide medical care, my mind began to wander as each triathlete crossed the finish line. Given my recent successes both with avoiding any sodium-related events in addition to my endurance accomplishments, I started to think that a triathlon may be my next logical progression. It had been mentioned to me previously, but my worries had always centered around the swim portion of a triathlon, which requires repeated, rapid head turning in order to breathe properly. By the end of that day though, having watched the elation in hundreds and hundreds of athletes as they crossed the finish line, I knew that a triathlon was my next goal.

Two weeks later, I purchased my first road bike. I began to swim – without incident – in our neighborhood pool. No Ménière's incidents. This gave me the confidence to push on – to swim harder, to bike faster and longer.

Eventually, the race arrived in April of 2016 and I felt ready, nervous as though I was. The swim portion of the race dominated my mind, but I was confident that if I could get through the swim I should be fine. Particularly concerning was that the swim would be taking place in the gulf, meaning that I would be swimming over a mile in salt water. As strange or trivial as it may sound to be worried about a saltwater swim triggering Ménière's, that is what the debilitating effects of Ménière's can do to one's mind. What if I swallowed small amounts of water repetitively throughout the swim? Would it add up to the same as drinking a glass of salt water? Would salt absorb through my skin? I had been working toward this goal for a year, and even though these concerns entered my mind, I pushed them down enough to finally be able to focus on the race.

Eventually, the race started. With no problems during the swim, I exited the water successfully. Similarly, I had no issues on the bike. And almost seven hours after starting my swim, I crossed the finish line of my first half-Ironman.

Triathlons come in many shapes and sizes. The short ones can be completed in well under two hours, while the grand Ironman series allows up to 17 hours for competitors to cross the finish line. Completing the half-Ironman had met my goal of conquering a triathlon, but soon I fell into the realization that I didn't have my next goal established. Once again my mind began to wander, and I knew that I would have to fill the void at some point.

Prior to almost every long race I entered I would get asked at some point why I signed up. Typically it was a non-runner, wondering somewhat facetiously why I would pay someone else money to run on a road, or even run at all. For most people, their quick answer was something along the lines of "a lifelong dream", or "to challenge myself". My reasons for entering a challenging race are far from these generic answers, and have a much more personal meaning.

For me, every time I cross a finish line it signifies another victory over Ménière's. Ménière's would win each time I dropped to the floor with vertigo, or canceled an event due to ongoing symptoms. Each time I cross the finish line after a race, I win. Every finished race is a celebration defying the price I had to pay during those years suffering from Ménière's. I don't enter races for the congratulations, or the swag, or to stand on a podium. I enter because I know the misery Ménière's once brought, and completing a race brings another accomplishment that during my Ménière's years I thought would never be possible. The second reason I enter these kinds of races is a bit simpler – if Ménière's ever returns in spite of my best efforts (i.e. maintaining my low-sodium diet), I want to be able to look back and know that I accomplished something during my days of being symptom-free.

Competing in these endurance events is somewhat contraindicated while on a low-sodium diet. Ask any endurance runner if salt is important during a race and you'll likely get a ten minute lecture on topics ranging from cramp prevention to electrolyte replacement. This belief explains why aid stations located throughout races are typically stocked with high-sodium foods such as potato chips, pretzels, and other snacks along with an abundance of salt packets similar to those you would find in the bottom of a fast food order. Some races even go so far as to have stations where volunteers hand out additional salt packets. For me, these were all to be avoided, limiting my sodium intake to that found in sports drinks and an occasional piece of fruit. Though this defies effectively every sports medicine and race nutrition protocol, when you are successful at holding back Ménière's, you will continue to do what has proven to work for you.

Going big time

A month after completing the half-Ironman I volunteered at a full Ironman held just a few miles from my house. Having completed the half-Ironman, I now considered myself a triathlete, and I was content with what I had accomplished. I had thrown around the idea that maybe a few years down the road, when my girls were a bit older, I would consider looking into completing a full Ironman. I had been incorrectly labeled an "Ironman" a couple of times over the past few weeks by a few friends. One unwritten rule about completing a half-Ironman is that finishers cannot call themselves an "Ironman", a moniker that holds a lot of weight for triathletes. That honor is saved for those who complete a full Ironman, consisting of 140.6 miles of swimming, biking, and running. Building up to my first half-Ironman I had no intent or desire to pursue earning the Ironman title. However, the string of accomplishments after having completed a half-marathon,

marathon, and half-Ironman needed to continue. Besides, stopping at "half" of anything isn't on any bucket list of mine.

By the end of that day working as a volunteer at the full Ironman, my next step would be set. Watching the participants cross the finish line in a range of emotional stages from sheer excitement to impassioned, doubled-over crying, I started to think of my own story. I wondered how many of these athletes have been where I've been – at a point so low that an event like an Ironman wasn't just a challenge, it was an absolute physical impossibility. From struggling to maintain my balance to completing 140.6 miles of endurance? The story writes itself, I thought. Why should I wait a few years to prove how far I've come? By the end of my finish-line shift I had decided that the next year I would be crossing the finish line, not watching others cross it.

A few weeks later I cautiously asked my wife if I could invest in a carbon triathlon bike, to which she wholeheartedly approved. And with that, my 10 month journey to becoming an Ironman began. I added a few more half-distance triathlons and two marathons over the next ten months, each of which were completed without any real reminder of the Ménière's.

With the longest endurance event of my life approaching, I started to wonder if my body was going to be able to maintain an adequate activity level in the presence of restricted sodium. I started to wonder if perhaps a marathon or half Ironman may be putting me right at the limit of entering into hyponatremia (low blood sodium), and whether a full Ironman might push me over the limit and leave me cramped, delusional, and needing medical treatment. I found myself wishing that I'd had my sodium levels measured prior to switching to a low-sodium diet in order to know if I was operating at any kind of deficit, or whether my values were within the normal range. Granted, with no concerns about sodium intake nor any blood work performed prior to my Ménière's attack I had no real reason to know or care about my sodium levels. But after having been on a restricted sodium diet and competing in endurance activities I became curious as to how my body had adapted to the reduced sodium diet. In October of 2016 I decided to perform a quasi-experiment to reveal a little insight into what was going on.

I was scheduled for my first-ever annual physical, so I ate my normal dinner the night before in order to prepare for my fasting blood draw the next morning. That morning, I got up early and ran my usual eight miles on a relatively humid morning. Afterwards, I avoided all fluids and food prior to my 10am appointment. I didn't want to influence my sodium value by diluting my body fluids, nor consume any additional sodium that would influence any of the other blood measures. The next day, my blood results came back. With a reference range of 135-146mEq/L, my sodium value came in squarely at . . . 143. Right within the 'normal' range, even leaning a bit toward the higher end of the scale after years of a low-sodium diet, after a sweaty 70-minute run, and no sodium consumption for the previous 13 hours.

Though the blood sodium value doesn't tell the whole story, it embraces much of what I believe – that sodium intake these days is much higher than what is required. On one hand, I was able to complete a long run with no effect on my blood sodium levels; on the other, my body had been used to a reduced-sodium intake and may have made adaptations to account for the lower sodium intake. However, total sodium lost via sweat depends on factors like sweat rate, sweat sodium content, humidity level, and other factors, and because I didn't measure my levels prior to running I don't know if my values went up, down, or stayed the same as a result of sweat loss. But it does provide intriguing information into a relationship between exercise and reduced-sodium intake, and I think that more research needs to be done. This is not to say that anyone should replicate my little experiment. In fact, no one should ever exercise without adequate replacement of fluids and electrolytes during and immediately after exercise, as doing so could be quite dangerous.

Finally, the day of the race arrived. A 4am alarm was no deterrent given the excitement and nerves that were running rampant. Arriving on site, adrenaline kicked in quickly. The pre-race ambiance at an Ironman event is addictive. The sight of almost 3,000 expensive bikes packed tightly together, the smell of tramped, muddy grass, and the sound of hushed enthusiasm serve to ramp up your excitement quickly. As I entered the water with visibility so bad that I couldn't even see my hand during each swim stroke, I started to wonder how I was going to survive the next 14, 15, 16, or 17 hours. Assuming that I would finish, of course. But I had to finish, because I didn't want to wait another year to try this again. Another year of training, of dreading the very swim event that I was participating in right now. If I can just survive for 90 minutes, the swim would be over. Over forever, I thought.

Faster than I expected, the swim was done. Now, on to the bike phase which I had dreamed about. Being on the bike meant that I had survived the swim, and as I hopped on my bike I felt almost like I had already accomplished my Ironman. I rationalized that anyone can ride a bike and run a marathon, but not everyone can survive a 2.4 mile swim. I did, and I didn't drown – so barring an equipment failure I didn't foresee anything stopping me. For the bike, I just needed to count to 112 very slowly – each number changing as I crossed another mile marker.

As I finished the bike, sore but undaunted, I realized that I was two-thirds of the way to my biggest goal yet. Now, it was just a slow count to 26 which I had done in several previous marathons. I had survived so far with no Ménière's events, and calculated that even if I got dizzy at some point, I had enough time remaining to take a rest break and still finish the race.

Eventually, as I approached the last few miles of the run portion, I thought back to my mindset for entering this race. I had completed a half-marathon, but had a couple of incidents to remind me that Ménière's was still lurking. Completing a marathon without incident allowed me to give a double-fisted middle finger to Ménière's. But the accomplishment of completing an Ironman – that deserves a much more violent, brutal assault on Ménière's.

As I hit mile 23, then mile 24, I started to think about what would happen in two miles when I crossed the finish line. I almost teared up twice just thinking of how I was going to cry at the finish line. No one else would understand why. They'd just see a middle-aged man crying at the end of his first Ironman like many other finishers and offer generic words of congratulations. But in my mind, finishing this race would signify victory over the most debilitating attacks I have ever been through. Victory over begging for sleep to come so that you could finally have some peace, only to have it contrasted with the anxiety that exists once awake. Victory over the three to four hours of helplessness during an attack combined with the 24 hours of constant angst brought about by waiting for the next attack. That's what my crying at the finish line would signify.

As I eventually turned onto the short uphill climb to the finish line and high-fived the crowd spilling over the barriers, a few short steps later it happened – I became an Ironman.

The excitement of the crowd in the last few hundred meters distracted me from releasing my emotions upon finishing the race. Hundreds of people lining the sides of the finish chute were screaming as each athlete crossed the finish line. Their enthusiasm drew me in, and I crossed the finish line with elation never once interrupted by emotion. I was lucky enough to have my wife and daughters at the race as well as my mom who had flown down to watch. The pride of completing a race many people train years for is something that stays with you a long time. For me, I consider it my proudest athletic accomplishment. So energizing was the emotion of finishing my first Ironman, as soon as the registration opened for the following year's race, I signed up.

Finishing the Ironman capped a nearly five year journey for me since my most brutal Ménière's attack. Once diagnosed with Ménière's, I had originally been somewhat frustrated with the fact that it wasn't curable and required a major lifestyle change to keep it under control. Over time, I was able to realize that the low sodium treatment method effectively eliminated my symptoms. I still have reminders every now and then. A few even stop me in my tracks for a split second. But no symptoms approach the severity and brutality of the attacks. Because of my adherence to a very low-sodium diet, for every birthday that my oldest daughter celebrates, I celebrate my own little anniversary of being attack-free. And because my girls have a lot of recitals, school events, and sports to participate in, I will continue to do what I need to do to ensure that I have many, many more anniversaries.

Chapter 8
Treatment of Ménière's

THERE IS CURRENTLY NO cure for Ménière's. As such, the next best option is to eliminate or at best control those symptoms associated with the disease. Many treatments are available ranging from simple lifestyle adaptations to surgical intervention. Typically, the course of treatment follows a plan which starts with the least involved (e.g. diet modification) and progresses through increasingly involved treatments until a favorable response occurs. Despite no cure for Ménière's, the success of medical intervention for Ménière's patients is favorable. Particularly encouraging is that 95% of patients report that vertigo attacks can be controlled with conservative medical management[28].

Whereas the symptoms of Ménière's can fluctuate in severity and even subside for months or years at a time, treatments are not consistent across patients. Furthermore, many patients often do not seek treatment until they are highly symptomatic[29], preventing early treatment options from lessening the impact of the disease. The lack of an accurate tool to assess the current stage of Ménière's in individual patients necessitates that all patients receive tailored treatment plans coordinated with their physician. Therefore, patients must work with their physician to outline the treatment plan best suited to their individual Ménière's situation.

At present, none of the available Ménière's treatments have been proven to stop or alter the natural progression of Ménière's. However, given the significant effect that Ménière's has on patient quality of life[30], any treatment which lessens the debilitating symptoms of Ménière's should be considered worthwhile. This chapter serves to review many of the most common treatments for Ménière's, from most conservative to most invasive.

Dietary and lifestyle changes

Sodium

Reducing sodium intake is typically the first option used in the treatment of Ménière's. Most Americans consume around 3,400mg of sodium per day, much higher than the Food and Drug Administration's recommendation of 2,300mg per day. Ménière's patients are typically recommended to reduce their sodium intake to 2000mg or even 1000mg under the direction of their physician. However, despite reported success with sodium reduction for the treatment of Ménière's the practice is not backed by scientific evidence. Furthermore, the mechanism by which sodium reduction improves Ménière's symptoms for some patients is not well understood.

Recent evidence suggests that it is not adherence to a low sodium diet that improves Ménière's symptoms as much as ensuring a constant sodium level within the body[21]. Because a Ménière's patient likely has a diminished ability to control fluid levels within the ear, a sharp spike in sodium can cause unregulated fluid fluctuations in the inner ear. Therefore, even a higher-than-recommended daily sodium intake of 2000-2500mg – when maintained at as constant of a level as possible – may prevent fluctuations in body sodium levels often associated with Ménière's attacks. Along with sodium intake, Ménière's patients should also

Mark Knoblauch

pay attention to events that *eliminate* sodium, such as profuse perspiration and diuretic use[21].

Caffeine

Caffeine is generally recommended to be eliminated from the diets of Ménière's patients. However, research indicates that the recommendation to restrict caffeine is largely anecdotal in nature and is not supported by evidence[31]. Interestingly, recent evidence indicates that Ménière's sufferers ingested caffeine at a much higher rate than non-Ménière's patients[32]. This is not to indicate caffeine as a cause of Ménière's; rather, it indicates a relationship may exist between caffeine use and Ménière's.

Surprisingly, a mechanistic reason for Ménière's patients to limit caffeine intake has not been clearly established. The rationale for limiting caffeine is limited, but has been mentioned to be linked to a vasoconstrictive effect of caffeine[33]. At present, strong evidence does not support the recommendation for Ménière's patients to reduce caffeine intake, yet the recommendation continues.

Other lifestyle factors

Along with sodium and caffeine reduction, several additional lifestyle factors have been reported to aggravate Ménière's symptoms. Alcohol consumption, smoking, and even chocolate and cheese consumption have been reported to increase Ménière's symptoms[34]. Unfortunately, most of these triggers are anecdotal in nature and lack research evidence confirming a consistent link between their use and Ménière's symptoms. Rather, these less common triggers often result from patients reporting an increase in Ménière's symptoms after associating with these triggers, yet fail to isolate their symptoms to one particular factor. Nevertheless, it is important for Ménière's patients to report any increase in symptoms to their doctor in order to determine their own unique triggers. Utilizing a diary, journal, or other record and detailing events occurring prior to an increase in Ménière's symptoms can be beneficial in establishing these primary triggers. And, as lifestyle triggers are identified, it may help reduce the frequency of Ménière's symptoms.

Medication

Pharmaceutical intervention is another non-invasive option for Ménière's treatment. Drugs used for Ménière's typically focus on either the removal of sodium from the blood (e.g. diuretics) or improvement of blood flow around the ear (e.g. betahistine). Like most lifestyle modifications, pharmaceutical treatment of Ménière's reports mixed success.

Diuretics

Diuretics focus predominantly on the removal of sodium from the body, which is thought to favorably alter endolymph electrolyte concentrations within the inner ear. This in turn reduces endolymph volume and pressure within the ear. In the United States, simultaneous use of hydrochlorothiazide and triamterene remains the drug treatment of choice for Ménière's[35]. However, a review of the medical literature reported that no quality studies warrant the use of diuretics for the treatment of Ménière's[36]. Still, combining diuretic therapy with reduced sodium intake has shown to slow the rate of hearing loss in Ménière's patients[37], and maintenance of hearing may help improve quality of life.

Betahistine

Betahistine is a drug that has shown to increase blood flow within the cochlea[38], but this benefit was shown to occur in guinea pigs and has not been corroborated in humans. Like diuretics, betahistine does not have strong support favoring its use, though its potential has been recognized and the need for further clinical trials has been outlined[39, 40]. Consequently, betahistine is not approved for the treatment of Ménière's in the United States despite having approval in Canada and Europe.

Suppressants

The third type of drug used in the treatment of Ménière's are the vestibular suppressant medications. Drugs such as benzodiazepines, meclizine, phenergan, scopolamine, and antihistamines fall into this class of Ménière's pharmaceutical treatment. These drugs are used to suppress the vestibular system during a Ménière's attack in an attempt to minimize or eliminate the accompanying vertigo symptoms. Because the drugs are used during an acute attack, complications can arise regarding their use. First, the drugs must be immediately available in the event that the vertigo limits the patient's ability to retrieve the drug. Second, the time required for the consumed drug to get taken up into the circulation and reach the target tissue can take hours, in turn reducing the overall effectiveness of these medications. Furthermore, the use of vestibular suppressant medications only affects those symptoms associated with an acute attack and have shown no benefit in slowing the progression of Ménière's.

Homeopathic treatment

Though not necessarily a medication, homeopathic methods are widely used for the treatment of Ménière's. To understand just how prevalent homeopathic treatment is, conduct a simple internet search for *homeopathic Ménière's*. You will get a wealth of treatment options ranging from chininum sulph to gelsemium to the *John of Ohio* regimen. Because of the vast amount of homeopathic treatment options available, they will not be detailed individually in this book. Ménière's patients should understand that many of these homeopathic treatments are anecdotal at best and have little to no scientific validity in the treatment of Ménière's. Patients must also be aware of misleading claims associated with homeopathic treatments as well as individuals who are out to take advantage of patients who are desperate for treatment. Of particular importance is that minimal – if any – quality research has been done on many of the recommended treatments and doses to establish data outlining interactions, dosing schedules, or efficacy. Still, a careful review of the medical literature will show that many of the well-researched Ménière's treatments (e.g. low-sodium adherence) have themselves shown little effect. As such, patients who have not responded to traditional Ménière's treatment may wish to consider homeopathic options after consulting with their physician.

Intra-tympanic injection

Injection of a substance through the eardrum is a typical course of action after conservative treatment such as lifestyle modifications and drug therapy measures have failed. By injecting through the eardrum rather than using oral or intravenous drug delivery, a dose can reach the target tissue quickly with fewer side effects. In fact, steroids injected into the middle ear can reach the perilymph within minutes[41].

Corticosteroids

For those patients whose vertigo attacks do not respond to the conservative treatment listed above, corticosteroids are often the next step in seeking relief from the attacks. Corticosteroids have several advantages including relatively easy application, supplying an anti-inflammatory dose directly to the inner ear, and not destroying any inner ear structure, thereby helping to preserve the hearing of affected patients[42]. Because the inner ear's *round window* membrane can allow certain drugs to pass through, intra-tympanic injection of steroids such as dexamethasone can reach the perilymph directly[43] and can result in up to a nearly 1.3-fold higher steroid concentration into the perilymph than systemic (i.e. oral, intravenous) delivery[44].

While an effective delivery method, intra-tympanic corticosteroid injections only serve to reduce the frequency of vertigo attacks for a relatively short (i.e. months) time period but do not stop nor reduce future attacks after the medication's effective window of six to eight months passes[45]. Consequently, multiple injections are often required.

Upon reviewing three individual studies that used intra-tympanic steroids, one set of researchers reported that there is viable evidence to support intra-tympanic steroid use such as dexamethasone for the treatment of Ménière's. However, the authors cautioned that more clarification is needed specific to the dose and frequency needed for successful treatment[42]. Along with dexamethasone, methylprednisolone is often used for intra-tympanic treatment of Ménière's[42]. It is thought that methylprednisolone can attain higher concentrations within the perilymph of the inner ear, allowing for potentially greater anti-inflammatory effects to be reached as a result of the higher drug concentration[46]. Furthermore, methylprednisolone has a greater binding affinity for mineralocorticoid receptors of the ear, which can influence hearing[47]. Still, some research suggests that dexamethasone is more successful in the treatment of Ménière's[48].

Gentamicin

Intra-tympanic injection of gentamicin into the inner ear has a much different mechanism than methylprednisolone or dexamethasone. While corticosteroid drugs are designed to reduce inflammation, gentamicin is an antibiotic that is actually toxic to nerves of the ear. Specifically, gentamicin targets vestibular hair cells, and intra-tympanic delivery of gentamicin allows it to enter the labyrinth and destroy hair cells in the semicircular canals of the affected ear. Although gentamicin targets hair cells, conflicting reports on the impact on patient's hearing have been reported to be both unaffected[29] and slightly diminished[49] after intra-tympanic gentamicin administration.

A more recent treatment method for gentamicin therapy is to begin intra-tympanic injections at a low dose initially, after which the dose is slowly increased to the point where vestibular deficits begin to show[50]. In terms of effectiveness, a recent review of the available literature reported that gentamicin can be effective in controlling vertigo in Ménière's patients[42]. However, given the potential impact on hearing, it was recommended that corticosteroid treatment is used initially. One study which directly compared gentamicin versus corticosteroids reported better control of vertigo in the gentamicin group two years after treatment than the corticosteroid group[49].

Surgical intervention

Invasive surgery for Ménière's generally falls into one of two categories – repair or ablation (i.e. destruction). Whereas ablation of any related organ can have severe consequences it is often the last resort in treatment of Ménière's. Unfortunately, when all other treatment options fail and the debilitating vertigo attacks remain it is often the only option available to the patient. Because of the relative complexity and sensitivity of each surgical procedure, surgery is typically reserved until after more conservative therapies have failed. It should also be noted that surgical destructive procedures are rarely performed these days, as other treatments (e.g. gentamicin) can be tailored to have a similar effect with much less cost and risk to the patient[29].

Endolymphatic sac shunt insertion or decompression

In a healthy ear, fluid should flow to the endolymph sac through the endolymphatic duct which is located inside of the vestibular aqueduct. When endolymph cannot flow normally through the aqueduct due to an event such as blockage, endolymphatic hydrops form. With endolymphatic sac shunt insertion surgery, a shunt (i.e. drain) is placed into the sac which in turn allows fluid to drain into the local bony area.

Endolymphatic decompression involves removal of bone surrounding the endolymph area. By doing so, any potential swelling of the endolymphatic sac is not inhibited by bone and as such the pressure does not increase within the sac. Because the endolymphatic sac is left intact, like endolymphatic shunt placement, endolymphatic sac decompression is not considered destructive in nature. Despite its nearly ninety years of use, research into the effectiveness of surgical manipulation of the endolymphatic sac remains somewhat inconclusive. In fact, some consider endolymphatic sac manipulation useless[51].

Vestibular Nerve Section

When non-destructive interventions fail to cease a Ménière's patient's incapacitating vertigo attacks, he or she is often left with the option of destroying the problematic nerve or organ that is likely triggering the attacks. For patients who have some level of hearing in the affected ear, sectioning (i.e. 'cutting') of the vestibular nerve can retain hearing despite effectively removing balance function in the ear.

When more conservative approaches fail to eliminate vertigo symptoms, vestibular nerve sectioning can eliminate those symptoms in approximately 95-98% of Ménière's patients[52]. Depending on the sectioning technique used, many patients will have an initial increase in vertigo that quickly subsides within days[53]. Though complications have been reported after the sectioning procedure, improvement in approaches used to section the nerve have reduced many postoperative complications[54].

Labyrinthectomy

Like vestibular nerve sectioning, labyrinthectomy results in the destruction of inner ear tissue. Unfortunately, labyrinthectomy also removes hearing function in the affected ear; therefore it is typically preferred for patients with no effective hearing in the ear affected by Ménière's[29]. After labyrinthectomy, elimination of vertigo can reach 97%[55].

Unfortunately, quality of life can be impacted if the body does not compensate for the loss of the affected ear's equilibrium organs. For example, postural instability can occur which is worsened by walking or moving. Post-labyrinthectomy disequilibrium incidence can reach as high as 78%, much higher than the 20% reported after vestibular neurectomy[54]. However, post-operative vestibular physical therapy can assist with improving quality of life[29].

Chapter 9
Medical Conditions Presenting Similar to Ménière's

IT IS IMPORTANT TO understand that Ménière's is a condition of exclusion, meaning that you can only be diagnosed with Ménière's after all other possible medical conditions have been excluded. Because the symptoms of Ménière's often mimic other related diseases, it is important that patients provide a clear medical history along with an exhaustive list of symptoms to their physician in order that he or she has the information necessary to make a quality diagnosis. Because vertigo and dizziness can be indicative of a range of diseases, this chapter serves to outline several conditions which can present symptoms similar to Ménière's.

Patients suffering from dizziness should understand that they are not alone – over one-third of Americans will seek medical care for dizziness in their lifetime[56]. It is important to point out that dizziness – as well as vertigo – are merely symptoms, and medical practitioners will first look for an underlying cause of each symptom rather than treating the actual symptom. In some cases, dizziness can be due to a condition as minor as dehydration. Other times, it can be more involved such as a cardiac condition. Despite the vast array of potential causes, this chapter will focus on those conditions which are similar to Ménière's in that they trigger dizziness and/or vertigo as a result of inner ear maladies.

Benign positional paroxysmal vertigo

One of the most common vertigo conditions seen in primary care is benign positional paroxysmal vertigo (BPPV)[57]. Despite the long name, each word plays a role in describing what occurs with the condition. Most patients with this relatively harmless (benign) condition describe sudden (paroxysmal) bouts of vertigo that occur with certain (positional) head positions.

The mechanism involved in BPPV is thought to be due to the presence of loose crystals (i.e. otoliths) within the semicircular canals of the ear. As otoliths are not normally present within the semicircular canals, certain head movements cause the loose otoliths to contact the delicate hair cells of the semicircular canal, causing them to trigger and falsely indicate body motion when the head is in particular positions. For example, patients with BPPV often report short bouts of vertigo when looking upwards or rolling over in bed[58]. Occasionally, nausea and vomiting can occur.

Diagnosis of BPPV typically involves a thorough medical history and evaluation along with manipulating the head in an attempt to reproduce the symptoms. Most commonly, the Dix-Hallpike maneuver is used to attempt to reproduce the symptoms of BPPV. For this procedure, the patient is seated on a table and head position is manipulated while the patient is put through a series of specific positions. Because the otoliths will typically induce nystagmus along with vertigo, the patient's eyes are observed for nystagmus in addition to any report of vertigo. Results of the Dix-Hallpike test are relatively reliable, being able to correctly identify patients with BPPV 83% of the time while correctly excluding patients without BPPV 52% of the time[57].

For those patients testing positive for BPPV, vestibular rehabilitation and canalith repositioning (e.g. the Epley maneuver) are relatively successful. Vestibular rehabilitation typically consists of a series of head and/or body motions which may involve fixation of the eye on a single point. Pharmaceutical treatments are not recommended for use in the treatment of BPPV as research has shown no benefit[59]. It is also possible that BBPV symptoms return.

Vestibular neuritis

Vestibular neuritis is associated with vertigo, nausea, vomiting, and imbalance, and is thought to be due to viral inflammation of the vestibular nerve[60]. The condition is acute in nature with symptoms lasting from a few days to several weeks, but up to half of those suffering from vestibular neuritis can experience symptoms much longer[61]. Vestibular neuritis has been reported to account for nearly 10% of all dizziness-related medical visits[62]. Interestingly, viral epidemics trigger an increased incidence of vestibular neuritis, lending evidence to its likely inflammatory origins.

Patients exhibiting vestibular neuritis will present with acute, severe vertigo[58]. The most severe attacks can last for one to two days and then gradually subside over the following weeks. Motion may worsen the vertigo, and some patients experience nausea and vomiting in conjunction with the vertigo[58]. Additional symptoms often include nystagmus as well as a walking pattern in which the patient tends to lean toward the affected ear's side.

Treatment of vestibular neuritis includes symptomatic care along with vestibular rehabilitation, which can begin as soon as tolerable after cessation of immediate symptoms[58]. Vestibular rehabilitation has been reported to be successful when compared against no therapy[63]. If vestibular neuritis is severe, short-term hospitalization may be required[58].

Vestibular migraine

Vestibular migraines are among the more common vestibular disorders, affecting up to 1% of the population[62, 64] and up to 11% of patients seeking treatment in dizziness-related clinics[65]. Vestibular migraines are also relatively common in children, having been reported to occur in nearly 3% of children aged 6-12 years of age[66]. Like Ménière's disease, vestibular migraine has no universally accepted definition which can in turn limit recognition of vestibular migraines in affected patients. Only recently were the diagnostic criteria established which include the following[65]:

1. Vestibular migraine
A. At least five episodes with vestibular symptoms of moderate or severe intensity, lasting from five minutes to 72 hours
B. A current or previous history of migraine with or without aura according to the International Classification of Headache Disorders (ICHD)
C. One or more migraine features with at least 50% of the vestibular episodes:
– a headache with at least two of the following characteristics: one sided location, pulsating quality, moderate or severe pain intensity, or aggravation by routine physical activity
– photophobia and phonophobia
– visual aura
D. Not better accounted for by another vestibular or ICHD diagnosis

2. Probable vestibular migraine
A. At least 5 episodes with vestibular symptoms of moderate or severe intensity, lasting five min to 72 hours
B. Only one of the criteria B and C for vestibular migraine is fulfilled (migraine history or migraine features during the episode)

C. Not better accounted for by another vestibular or ICHD diagnosis

The predominant symptoms of vestibular migraine include vertigo in combination with a headache, and these two symptoms often occur relatively close to each other[58]. Other symptoms can include transient hearing fluctuations[67], nausea, vomiting, and a sensitivity to motion sickness[65]. Some patients have reported triggering of their migraine in response to dehydration, lack of sleep, or certain foods, but the relationship between these characteristics and vestibular migraines has not been well-studied[65].

Evidence of effective treatment of vestibular migraines is limited. Patients who respond favorably to anti-migraine medication have occurred, but the evidence is lacking as to overall effectiveness[68].

Chapter 10
Ménière's and Quality of Life

I F YOU HAVE MÉNIÈRE'S, you know that life can be miserable. And when life is miserable, your own quality of life diminishes. Having now read the chapter outlining my own experience with Ménière's, you are aware how Ménière's dominated my thoughts, affected my decisions, and largely determined my daily schedule. Not knowing if I would be incapacitated for three hours during the attack – plus the following two to three hours of sleep – at any random point during the day caused me extreme, ongoing anxiety. As I outlined, I felt as if I were a prisoner in my own body as I was constrained by the constant chance that a full attack could occur. And if one didn't occur, the random and sometimes forceful symptoms led me to feel as though an attack was imminent.

The research on Ménière's-related quality of life is not consistent. This may stem in part from a sort of 'chicken and egg' quandary in that it is not clear as to whether a psychological condition comes first or the disease is the initial culprit[69]. Regardless, there is little argument that the effects of the disease are quite significant.

For example, survey results led one group of researchers to conclude that " . . . Ménière's seems to be one of the most debilitating diseases experienced by people who survive any illness"[70], a statement that I would guess will be agreed with by many Ménière's sufferers. Another study found that nearly two-thirds of Ménière's patients suffer from anxiety and depression, and that those patients who have had the disease the longest suffered more stressors, worse social and physical functioning, and reported more pain than those suffering for less time[71]. However, a separate study of Ménière's patients treated surgically versus non-surgically found that most patients self-rated their quality of life as "good" or "very good"[72]. This conflicting research strengthens the notion that every patient's symptoms are different, which transfers over to perceived quality of life as well.

It should be noted that research indicates that some of the negative quality of life is brought about by the stress of Ménière's itself. Stress hormones have been shown to be elevated in patients with conditions involving endolymphatic hydrops such as Ménière's. Researchers suspected that the elevated hormones altered the ability of the inner ear to regulate fluid, in turn producing symptoms of Ménière's[73]. This would suggest that Ménière's indeed generates a vicious cycle in that the disease causes stress and the stress aggravates the disease, certainly a problem for Ménière's sufferers who are affected psychologically by the effects of the disease.

Unpredictable vertigo has consistently been reported as the biggest physical determinant of reduced quality of life[74-76]. In fact, among both Ménière's and non-Ménière's patients, disabling vertigo has been implicated as the symptom most likely to cause mental disorders[77]. The vertigo associated with Ménière's has been reported to cause certain daily activities to become difficult such as driving, using ladders, or climbing stairs[78]. This in turn caused anxiety towards situations perceived as potential triggers for an attack which included travel, heights, stress, or anger, among others. Furthermore, as Ménière's progresses over time, tinnitus and reduced hearing have reported as becoming increasingly detrimental to quality of life[75].

Psychologic factors that may predispose an individual to Ménière's have been examined. As a Ménière's patient might hope, research has found no abnormal personality traits in Ménière's patients[71]. In fact, one study reported that Ménière's patients typically have a specific personality that includes high intelligence, diligence, and a strong sense of duty[79]. This finding was countered by another study that conveyed Ménière's patients as obsessive-compulsive perfectionists as well as a bit neurotic, and who would be considered vulnerable and more exposed to stress. However, those same researchers concluded that any psychological characteristics of Ménière's are generally due to Ménière's rather than responsible for causing Ménière's itself[80]. For those psychological conditions associated with Ménière's, psychotherapy has been shown effective at improving coping mechanisms along with reducing symptoms of depression and anxiety associated with Ménière's[81].

In order to target factors that influence quality of life, evaluating all symptoms associated with Ménière's can help identify those specific symptoms that have the biggest influence on quality of life. In order to capture data that can be used to evaluate quality of life, surveys can be beneficial. In fact, two dedicated Ménière's-based surveys have been around for more than a decade: the Ménière's Disease Outcome Questionnaire and the Ménière's Disease-Patient Oriented Survey Index, but results from these studies must be interpreted with caution as the surveys have not yet been validated[82]. More recently, the Ménière's Disease Disability Scale was developed in 2017 to determine quality of life for patients with Ménière's, with promising results[82]. Further development of Ménière's-specific surveys is important as effective surveys can generate data that can reveal particular insights into the effects of Ménière's.

As discussed throughout this book, the quality of life of Ménière's patients has been improved through lifestyle modifications including a reduction in sodium as well as through various treatment (e.g. vestibular rehabilitation) or intratympanic or surgical options. For me, strict control of my sodium has been the only treatment needed up to this point; yet, given the course that Ménière's can take over the long-term, I am cognizant that my condition may worsen over time and require additional treatment. If you have experienced a reduced quality of life as a result of your Ménière's, know that you are not alone. As we have outlined in this chapter, quality of life is diminished to some degree for many Ménière's patients compared to a healthy population. This should not be unexpected in a disease in which over half of sufferers report never being free of discomfort resulting from Ménière's[75]. Given the vast range and degree of symptoms, it is critical that you seek treatment for not only the physical symptoms of Ménière's but also for any psychological effects that so often accompany this disease.

Chapter 11
In Conclusion . . .

A S YOU HAVE READ throughout this book, Ménière's is a
highly involved and highly variable disease. Both the
overwhelming effects of the disease along with the
complexity of the symptoms are largely what pushed me towards
writing this book. It's easy to explain how flu symptoms bother
you or how a sore shoulder feels, as pretty much everyone has had
similar symptoms. However, the internal, vestibular-focused
symptoms associated with Ménière's are much more complicated.
During my symptomatic years, I often grew frustrated as I was
conflicted by wanting to talk about what I was going through, yet
at the same time knowing that no one would *really* understand
outside of a lending a compassionate ear. In writing this book I felt
that by detailing my experiences, Ménière's patients could know
that someone truly understands what they are going through, and
those who interact with someone who has the disease can perhaps
better understand what that person is dealing with.

The second reason for writing this book stems from the
success that I have had in effectively eliminating my Ménière's
symptoms after having adhered to a low-sodium lifestyle. I had
resigned myself to living with Ménière's the rest of my life, and
given the fact that there was no cure, I accepted and firmly

believed that I was never going to get better. But, I got better. And better. And now I consider myself effectively Ménière's free. Yes, there are still little reminders that occur every now and then, but those events happen far less than 1% of the time. That's why I say that I am "effectively" or "almost" Ménière's free. I still have tinnitus (a symptom of Ménière's but also a condition all by itself), I still grip the steering wheel a little harder if I hit a wavy spot in the road, and I still have split-second bits of unsteadiness every now and then if I turn a corner too quickly. But for the most part, Ménière's is not a part of my life. If you are living with Ménière's, this book was written to give you hope that a solution may exist for you the same way it did for me.

I hope that this book has been informative for you. In writing it, I have learned a great deal more about Ménière's than I knew previously, and I encourage you to also continue to expand your knowledge of this debilitating disease. As Ménière's research continues to expand, new therapies and treatments are likely to follow close behind, allowing us to advance toward finding a cure for this disease. And when it comes to your own treatment, know that if one treatment does not work, you must move on to the next. Statistically speaking, you are going to get relief from treatment – you just have to press on until you find the treatment that is successful for you. Work carefully with your physician and keep him or her updated as to your progress so that you can adjust or maintain treatments as needed. Be wary of potential scams relating to treatments and devices, yet remain open to the possibility of new discoveries that can help. In the meantime, look into the many online options (e.g. associations, forums, medical sites, etc.,) that can help provide you information as well as support.

Finally, I wish you the best of treatments to you in your continued journey with Ménière's.

Glossary

Ablation: surgical removal of body tissue

Action potential: the transmission of a signal along a cell membrane that results from manipulation of charged ions

Anterior canal: one of the semicircular canals that is responsible for detecting motion of the head such as occurs when nodding one's head to indicate "yes"

Cochlea: the organ of the inner ear shaped like a snail's shell which is responsible for receiving vibrations from the eardrum and converting them into electrical signals for transmission to the brain

Compound: a substance made up of two or more individual elements

Depolarization: the change in the resting electrical charge surrounding a cell membrane

Diuretic: a drug used to increase the removal of water and salt from the body

Dizziness: a sensation that results in the patient feeling as if he or she is spinning or moving while remaining stationary

Endolymph: the potassium-rich fluid contained within the membranous labyrinth of the ear

Endolymphatic Hydrops: a disorder of the inner ear's vestibular system resulting from abnormal accumulation of endolymph

Endolymphatic sac: a component of the inner ear membrane system filled with endolymph and thought to be involved in regulating the pressure as well as the volume of the endolymph

Equilibrium: a state of overall balance

Horizontal canal: one of the semicircular canals that is responsible for detecting motion of the head such as occurs when shaking one's head to indicate "no"

Inner Ear: the portion of the ear within the temporal bone that contains the semicircular canals and cochlea

Ion: a charged atom that has gained its charge due to the loss or gain of electrons

Ion channel: a passageway through a cell membraned formed by proteins and which allows specific ions to pass through

Ion pump: a membrane-embedded protein structure that moves ions across a cell membrane from an area of low concentration to an area of high concentration.

Ménière's Disease: a condition of the inner ear comprised of symptoms that include vertigo, tinnitus, hearing loss, and the sensation of ear fullness

Middle Ear: the central cavity of the inner ear comprised of the empty space within the temporal bone located inside of the eardrum

Milligram: a unit of weight, equivalent to $1/1000^{th}$ of a gram

Nutrition facts label: a required label found on the exterior of processed food packages that outlines various nutrition content of the food item as well as the serving size

Organ of Corti: an organ of the inner ear that is responsible for transmitting sound vibrations into nerve signals

Otolith: small calcium-based structures of the inner ear designed to assist with detecting head motion

Otolithic Membrane: the gelatinous portion of the inner ear that is embedded with otoliths and serves as a material that the ear can use to aid in the detection of head motion

Outer Ear: That portion of the ear that is visible, along with the auditory canal

Perilymph: a sodium-rich and potassium-poor fluid of the membranous labyrinth

Posterior canal: one of the semicircular canals that is responsible for detecting motion of the head such as occurs when placing an ear on its same-side shoulder

Resting potential: the electrical charge surrounding a cell membrane when at rest

Round window: the permeable membrane of the inner ear that allows fluid movement to occur in response to vibrations from the middle ear

Saccule: like the utricle, an area concentrated with sensory nerves with the inner ear and responsible for detecting head movement

Semicircular Canals: three fluid-filled tubes of the inner ear responsible for detecting head movement

Serving size: the portion of food or drink that is typically served

Sodium: a silver-white, highly volatile element

Tumarkin Falls: a condition in which individuals with inner-ear dysfunction experience a rapid onset of vertigo that results in the individual falling suddenly to the ground

Utricle: like the saccule, an area concentrated with sensory nerves with the inner ear and responsible for detecting head movement

Vertigo: a sensation of spinning that is usually accompanied by a sudden loss of balance

Vestibular aqueduct: a small, bone-encased canal that extends from the inner ear's endolymphatic space toward the brain

Vestibular nerve: the eighth cranial nerve, responsible for transmitting hearing and sensory information from the inner ear to the brain

References

1. Salt, A.N. and H. Rask-Andersen, *Responses of the endolymphatic sac to perilymphatic injections and withdrawals: evidence for the presence of a one-way valve.* Hearing research, 2004. **191**(1-2): p. 90-100.

2. Friberg, U., J. Stahle, and A. Svedberg, *The natural course of Meniere's disease.* Acta Oto-Laryngologica, 1983. **96**(sup406): p. 72-77.

3. Hart, C.W., *Meniere's disease: terminology and data bank acquisition.* The American journal of otology, 1981. **2**(3): p. 216-218.

4. Lopez-Escamez, J., et al., *Classification Committee of the Barany Society; Japan Society for Equilibrium Research; European Academy of Otology and Neurotology (EAONO); Equilibrium Committee of the American Academy of Otolaryngology-Head and Neck Surgery (AAO-HNS); Korean Balance Society. Diagnostic criteria for Menière's disease.* J Vestib Res, 2015. **25**(1): p. 1-7.

5. Baloh, R.W., *Prosper Meniere and his disease.* Archives of neurology, 2001. **58**(7): p. 1151-1156.

6. Hearing, C.o. and Equilibrium, *Committee on Hearing and Equilibrium guidelines for the diagnosis and evaluation of therapy in Meniere's disease.* Otolaryngology–Head and Neck Surgery, 1995. **113**(3): p. 181-185.

7. Pearson, B.W. and D.E. Brackmann, *Committee on hearing and equilibrium guidelines for reporting treatment*

results in Meniere's disease. 1985, SAGE Publications Sage CA: Los Angeles, CA.

8. Ishiyama, G., et al., *Meniere's disease: histopathology, cytochemistry, and imaging.* Annals of the New York Academy of Sciences, 2015. **1343**(1): p. 49-57.

9. Havia, M., E. Kentala, and I. Pyykko, *Prevalence of Menière's disease in general population of Southern Finland.* Otolaryngology–Head and Neck Surgery, 2005. **133**(5): p. 762-8.

10. Harris, J. and T. Alexander, *Current-day prevalence of Ménière's syndrome.* Audiology and neuro-otology, 2010. **15**(5): p. 318-22.

11. Alexander, T. and J. Harris, *Current epidemiology of Meniere's syndrome.* Otolaryngologic Clinics of North America, 2010. **43**(5): p. 965-70.

12. Minor, L., D. Schessel, and J. Carey, *Meniere's Disease.* Current Opinion in Neurology, 2004. **17**(1): p. 9-16.

13. Morita, N., et al., *Membranous labyrinth volumes in normal ears and Ménière disease: A three-dimensional reconstruction study.* The Laryngoscope, 2009. **119**(11): p. 2216-2220.

14. Schuknecht, H., ed. *Endolymphatic Hydrops.* 2nd ed. Pathology of the Ear. 1993, Lea and Febiger: Philadelphia.

15. Nakashima, T., et al., *Endolymphatic hydrops revealed by intravenous gadolinium injection in patients with Ménière's disease.* Acta oto-laryngologica, 2010. **130**(3): p. 338-343.

16. Merchant, S.N., J.C. Adams, and J.B. Nadol Jr, *Pathophysiology of Meniere's syndrome: are symptoms caused by endolymphatic hydrops?* Otology & Neurotology, 2005. **26**(1): p. 74-81.

17. Gurkov, R., et al., *In vivo visualization of endolyphatic hydrops in patients with Meniere's disease: correlation with audiovestibular function.* European Archives of Oto-Rhino-Laryngology, 2011. **268**(12): p. 1743-1748.

18. Sepahdari, A.R., et al., *Delayed intravenous contrast-enhanced 3D FLAIR MRI in Meniere's disease: correlation of quantitative measures of endolymphatic hydrops with hearing.* Clinical imaging, 2015. **39**(1): p. 26-31.

19. Calzada, A.P., et al., *Otolithic membrane damage in patients with endolymphatic hydrops and drop attacks.* Otology & neurotology: official publication of the American Otological Society, American Neurotology Society [and] European Academy of Otology and Neurotology, 2012. **33**(9): p. 1593.

20. Candreia, C., N. Schmuziger, and N. Gürtler, *Molecular analysis of aquaporin genes 1 to 4 in patients with Meniere's disease.* Cellular physiology and biochemistry, 2010. **26**(4-5): p. 787-792.

21. Rauch, S.D., *Clinical hints and precipitating factors in patients suffering from Meniere's disease.* Otolaryngologic Clinics of North America, 2010. **43**(5): p. 1011-1017.

22. angasniemi, E. and E. Hietikko, *The theory of autoimmunity in Meniere's disease is lacking evidence.* Auris Nasus Larynx, 2017.

23. Vrabec, J.T., *Herpes simplex virus and Meniere's disease.* The Laryngoscope, 2003. **113**(9): p. 1431-1438.

24. Bjorne, A., A. Berven, and G. Agerberg, *Cervical signs and symptoms in patients with Meniere's disease: a controlled study.* CRANIO®, 1998. **16**(3): p. 194-202.

25. Söderman, A.C.H., et al., *Stress as a Trigger of Attacks in Menière's Disease. A Case-Crossover Study.* The laryngoscope, 2004. **114**(10): p. 1843-1848.

26. Furstenberg, A., F. Lashmet, and F. Lathrop, *LXXXIV. Ménière's Symptom Complex: Medical Treatment.* 1934, SAGE Publications Sage CA: Los Angeles, CA.

27. Food and Drug Administration, *A Food Labeling Guide. Guidance For Industry.* 2013.

28. Colletti, V., M. Carner, and L. Colletti, *Auditory results after vestibular nerve section and intratympanic gentamicin*

for Ménière's disease. Otology & Neurotology, 2007. **28**(2): p. 145-151.

29. Sharon, J., et al., *Treatment of Ménière's Disease.* Current Treatment Options in Neurology, 2015. **17**(4): p. 341.

30. Levo, H., et al., *Fatigue in Ménière's disease.* Hearing, Balance and Communication, 2013. **11**(4): p. 191-197.

31. Luxford, E., et al., *Dietary modification as adjunct treatment in Ménière's disease: Patient willingness and ability to comply.* Otology & Neurotology, 2013. **34**(8): p. 1438-1443.

32. Sánchez-Sellero, I., et al., *Caffeine intake and Ménière's disease: Is there relationship?* Nutritional neuroscience, 2017: p. 1-8.

33. Ledesma, A., ed. *Caffeine and Meniere's Disease.* Up to Date on Meniere's Disease, ed. F. Bahmad Jr. 2017, InTech.

34. Harcourt, J., K. Barraclough, and A.M. Bronstein, *Meniere's disease.* bmj, 2014. **349**: p. g6544.

35. Foster, C.A., *Optimal management of Ménière's disease.* Therapeutics and clinical risk management, 2015. **11**: p. 301.

36. Thirlwall, A. and S. Kundu, *Diuretics for Ménière's disease or syndrome.* The Cochrane Database of Systemic Reviews, 2006. **19**(3): p. CD003599.

37. Santos, P.M., et al., *Diuretic and diet effect on Meniere's disease evaluated by the 1985 Committee on Hearing and Equilibrium guidelines.* Otolaryngology—Head and Neck Surgery, 1993. **109**(4): p. 680-689.

38. Ihler, F., et al., *Betahistine exerts a dose-dependent effect on cochlear stria vascularis blood flow in guinea pigs in vivo.* PloS one, 2012. **7**(6): p. e39086.

39. Adrion, C., et al., *Efficacy and safety of betahistine treatment in patients with Meniere's disease: primary results of a long term, multicentre, double blind, randomised,*

placebo controlled, dose defining trial (BEMED trial). bmj, 2016. **352**: p. h6816.

40. James, A. and M.J. Burton, *Betahistine for Meniere's disease or syndrome.* The Cochrane Library, 2001.

41. Hargunani, C.A., et al., *Intratympanic injection of dexamethasone: time course of inner ear distribution and conversion to its active form.* Otology & Neurotology, 2006. **27**(4): p. 564-569.

42. Syed, M., et al., *Intratympanic therapy in Meniere's syndrome or disease: up to date evidence for clinical practice.* Clinical Otolaryngology, 2015. **40**(6): p. 682-690.

43. Garduño-Anaya, M.A., et al., *Dexamethasone inner ear perfusion by intratympanic injection in unilateral Meniere's disease: a two-year prospective, placebo-controlled, double-blind, randomized trial.* Otolaryngology-Head and Neck Surgery, 2005. **133**(2): p. 285-294.

44. Bird, P.A., et al., *Intratympanic versus intravenous delivery of methylprednisolone to cochlear perilymph.* Otology & Neurotology, 2007. **28**(8): p. 1124-1130.

45. Al Attrache, N.A., et al., *Response Over Time of Vertigo Spells to Intratympanic Dexamethasone Treatment in Meniere's Disease Patients.* J Int Adv Otol, 2016. **12**(1): p. 92-7.

46. Masoumi, E., et al., *Methylprednisolone versus Dexamethasone for Control of Vertigo in Patients with Definite Meniere's disease.* Iranian Journal of Otorhinolaryngology, 2017. **29**(95): p. 341.

47. Patel, M., et al., *Intratympanic methylprednisolone versus gentamicin in patients with unilateral Ménière's disease: a randomised, double-blind, comparative effectiveness trial.* The Lancet, 2016. **388**(10061): p. 2753-2762.

48. Hamid, M. and D. Trune, *Issues, indications, and controversies regarding intratympanic steroid perfusion.* Current opinion in otolaryngology & head and neck surgery, 2008. **16**(5): p. 434.

49. Casani, A., et al., *Intratympanic treatment of intractable unilateral Meniere disease: gentamicin or dexamethasone? A randomized controlled trial.* Otolaryngology-Head and Neck Surgery, 2012. **146**(3): p. 430-7.

50. Chia, S., et al., *Intratympanic gentamicin therapy for Meniere's disease: a meta-analysis.* Otology & Neurotology, 2004. **25**(4): p. 544-52.

51. Bretlau, P., et al., *Placebo effect in surgery for Menière's disease: nine-year follow-up.* The American journal of otology, 1989. **10**(4): p. 259-261.

52. Gacek, R.R. and M.R. Gacek, *Comparison of labyrinthectomy and vestibular neurectomy in the control of vertigo.* The Laryngoscope, 1996. **106**(2): p. 225-230.

53. Setty, P., et al., *Fully endoscopic retrosigmoid vestibular nerve section for refractory Meniere disease.* Journal of Neurological Surgery Part B: Skull Base, 2016. **77**(04): p. 341-349.

54. Alarcón, A.V., et al., *Labyrinthectomy and Vestibular Neurectomy for Intractable Vertiginous Symptoms.* International archives of otorhinolaryngology, 2017. **21**(02): p. 184-190.

55. Hammerschlag, P.E. and H.F. Schuknecht, *Transcanal labyrinthectomy for intractable vertigo.* Archives of Otolaryngology, 1981. **107**(3): p. 152-156.

56. Agrawal, Y., et al., *Disorders of balance and vestibular function in US adults: data from the National Health and Nutrition Examination Survey, 2001-2004.* Archives of internal medicine, 2009. **169**(10): p. 938-944.

57. Hanley, K., *Symptoms of vertigo in general practice: a prospective study of diagnosis.* Br J Gen Pract, 2002. **52**(483): p. 809-812.

58. Wipperman, J., *Dizziness and vertigo.* Primary Care: Clinics in Office Practice, 2014. **41**(1): p. 115-131.

59. Bhattacharyya, N., et al., *Clinical practice guideline: benign paroxysmal positional vertigo.* Otolaryngology--Head and Neck Surgery, 2008. 139(5_suppl): p. 47-81.

60. Schuknecht, H.F. and K. Kitamura, *Vestibular neuritis.* Annals of Otology, Rhinology & Laryngology, 1981. 90(1_suppl): p. 1-19.

61. Perols, J.B., Olle, *Vestibular neuritis: a follow-up study.* Acta oto-laryngologica, 1999. 119(8): p. 895-899.

62. Neuhauser, H.K. and T. Lempert. *Vertigo: epidemiologic aspects.* in *Seminars in neurology.* 2009. © Thieme Medical Publishers.

63. Hillier, S.L. and M. McDonnell, *Vestibular rehabilitation for unilateral peripheral vestibular dysfunction.* The Cochrane Library, 2011.

64. Cherchi, M. and T.C. Hain, *Migraine-associated vertigo.* Otolaryngologic Clinics of North America, 2011. 44(2): p. 367-375.

65. Lempert, T., et al., *Vestibular migraine: diagnostic criteria.* Journal of Vestibular Research, 2012. 22(4): p. 167-172.

66. Abu-Arafeh, I. and G. Russell, *Paroxysmal vertigo as a migraine equivalent in children: a population-based study.* Cephalalgia, 1995. 15(1): p. 22-25.

67. Johnson, G.D., *Medical Management of Migraine-Related Dizziness and Vertigo.* The Laryngoscope, 1998. 108(S85): p. 1-28.

68. Fotuhi, M., et al., *Vestibular migraine: a critical review of treatment trials.* Journal of neurology, 2009. 256(5): p. 711-716.

69. Orji, F., *The influence of psychological factors in Meniere's disease.* Annals of medical and health sciences research, 2014. 4(1): p. 3-7.

70. Anderson, J.P. and J.P. Harris, *Impact of Meniere's disease on quality of life.* Otology & neurotology, 2001. 22(6): p. 888-894.

71. Van Cruijsen, N., et al., *Psychological assessment of patients with Menière's disease: Evaluación psicológica de pacientes con enfermedad de Menière.* International journal of audiology, 2006. **45**(9): p. 496-502.

72. Söderman, A.-C.H., et al., *Patients' subjective evaluations of quality of life related to disease-specific symptoms, sense of coherence, and treatment in Meniere's disease.* Otology & neurotology, 2001. **22**(4): p. 526-533.

73. Juhn, S.K., et al., *Effect of stress-related hormones on inner ear fluid homeostasis and function.* American Journal of Otology, 1999. **20**(6): p. 800-806.

74. Erlandsson, S., M. Eriksson-Mangold, and A. Wiberg, *Ménière's disease: trauma, distress and adaptation studied through focus interview analyses.* Scandinavian audiology. Supplementum, 1996. **43**: p. 45-56.

75. Hägnebo, C., et al., *The influence of vertigo, hearing impairment and tinnitus on the daily life of Meniere patients.* Scandinavian audiology, 1997. **26**(2): p. 69-76.

76. Söderman, A.-C.H., et al., *Factors influencing quality of life in patients with Meniere's disease, identified by a multidimensional approach.* Otology & neurotology, 2002. **23**(6): p. 941-948.

77. Wexler, M. and W.G. Crary, *Meniere's disease: the psychosomatic hypothesis.* Otology & Neurotology, 1986. **7**(2): p. 93-96.

78. Yardley, L., B. Dibb, and G. Osborne, *Factors associated with quality of life in Meniere's disease.* Clinical Otolaryngology, 2003. **28**(5): p. 436-441.

79. Groen, J., *Psychosomatic aspects of Meniere's disease.* Acta oto-laryngologica, 1983. **95**(5-6): p. 407-416.

80. Savastano, M., et al., *Illness behaviour, personality traits, anxiety, and depression in patients with Ménière's disease.* The Journal of otolaryngology, 1996. **25**(5): p. 329-333.

81. Sterkers, O., et al., *Meniere's Disease 1999.* 1999: Kugler Publications.

82. Mutlu, B., et al., *The Reliability and Validity of "Dokuz Eylül University Meniere's Disease Disability Scale".* The journal of international advanced otology, 2017.

Image Credits

Figure 1.1: Ear structure: MedicalArtInc/shutterstock.com
Figure 1.2: Inner Ear: Maxcreatnz/shutterstock.com
Figure 1.3: Ear membranes: blamb/shutterstock.com
Figure 6.1: Nutrition Label: Jamie cross/shutterstock.com

Made in the USA
Las Vegas, NV
22 July 2021

26827987R00079